Heart conditions and treatments

By

Lucy R. Velazquez

Copyright@2023 by Lucy R. Velazquez

Table of Content

Introduction

Your heart is one of your body's most important organs. Essentially a pump, the heart is a muscle made up of four chambers separated by valves and divided into two halves. Each half contains one chamber called an atrium and one called a ventricle. The atria (plural for atrium) collect blood, and the ventricles contract to push blood out of the heart. The right half of the heart pumps oxygen-poor blood (blood that has a low amount of oxygen) to the lungs, where blood cells can obtain more oxygen. Then, the newly oxygenated blood travels from the lungs into the left atrium and the left ventricle. The left ventricle pumps the newly oxygen-rich blood to the organs and tissues of the body. This oxygen provides your body with energy and is essential to keeping your body healthy.

Heart condition and treatments

The general term used to cover malfunctions of the heart is heart disease, or sometimes cardiac disease ("Cardiac" is a Latin term for the heart). Though there are multiple forms of heart disease, our discussion focuses on the two most common: Heart attack and heart failure. This document is designed to teach you about heart attacks and heart failure: what causes these diseases, what forms these diseases take, and what can be done to treat these diseases when they occur. As both of these diseases are to some extent avoidable, we have also provided a discussion of preventative steps you can take to decrease your chances of having to deal with heart disease or to minimize the negative effects of existing heart disease. Although heart disease can occur in different forms, there is a common set of core risk factors that influence whether someone will ultimately be at risk for heart disease or not.

The goal of this book is to give a thorough explanation of heart disease, including its type, forms, causes, risk factors, symptoms, diagnosis, available treatments, and preventative actions.

Enjoy your time, unwind, and pay attention to these game-changing techniques.

Chapter 1

Heart disease definition and different forms of heart disease?

Heart disease, usually referred to as cardiovascular disease, is a general term for a number of heart-related ailments. It is a significant threat to world health and a leading cause of mortality and disability. For the prevention, diagnosis, and treatment of heart disease, it is essential to comprehend its complexities.

There are many different cardiac disorders that fall under the umbrella term "heart disease." Coronary artery disease (CAD), which impairs cardiac blood flow, is the most prevalent kind of heart disease in the US. A heart attack may result from reduced blood flow. The term "heart disease" refers to a variety of heart-related illnesses.

The following list of conditions is associated with heart disease:

- Abnormal cardiac rhythms (arrhythmias)

- Birth abnormalities of the heart (congenital heart defects)

- Heart muscle disease

- Heart valve illness

Healthy lifestyle choices can either prevent or treat many types of heart disease.

Heart disease is any ailment that compromises the heart's structure or functionality. Heart disease is typically considered an ailment. Heart disease, however, is actually a set of illnesses with a wide range of underlying causes.

Types of heart disease

There are many different types of heart disease. Some types can be grouped together according to how they affect the structure or

function of your
heart.

1. Coronary artery disease (CAD)

Coronary artery disease (CAD) is the most common form of heart disease. It occurs when one or more of the coronary arteries become narrow or blocked. Normally, blood flows through blood vessels like water through a hose. In coronary artery disease, major blood vessels that supply blood, oxygen, and nutrients to the heart become damaged or diseased. This damage causes the vessels to become narrow, stiff, or blocked. The process is often called hardening of the arteries, or atherosclerosis.

CAD may lead to:

- Angina (chest discomfort)

- (myocardial infarction) Heart attack

- Heart suddenly stopping (cardiac arrest)

Types

There are three types of coronary artery disease; they include:

1. Obstructive: Blood vessels have significantly narrowed or blocked.

2. Non-obstructive: Blood vessels have narrowed because they have branched off to smaller vessels or are due to the heart muscle squeezing too tightly on the vessels.

3. SCAD: Spontaneous coronary artery dissection (SCAD) refers to the tearing of blood vessels in the heart. Learn more about SCAD.

Who is at risk?

Risk factors for heart disease are conditions or habits that make it more likely that you will get heart disease. Some risk factors for coronary artery disease can be changed, and others cannot.

Risk factors you can change:

- high blood pressure
- High blood cholesterol and triglycerides
- diabetes
- unhealthy weight
- unhealthy diet
- too much alcohol
- not enough physical activity
- smoking or chewing tobacco
- stress
- depression

Risk factors you cannot change:

- Age: the older you are, the higher your risk of heart disease.
- **Sex:** Your risk of heart disease and stroke increases after menopause.
- Family history: if you have a close relative who has experienced heart

disease at an early age, you are at increased risk. In addition, women who have had pre-eclampsia during pregnancy have an increased risk.

- Indigenous heritage: First Nations, Metis, and Inuit peoples have a higher risk of heart disease than the general population. They are more likely to have high blood pressure (hypertension) and diabetes. Both conditions can cause heart disease.

- South Asian and African heritage: people of African or South Asian background have a higher risk of heart disease. They are more likely to have high blood pressure (hypertension), diabetes, or other risk factors for heart disease at a younger age.

- Personal circumstances: Personal circumstances and environmental factors have an influence on your health. This includes things such as access to healthy food, safe drinking water, health services, and social services.

Causes

Over many years, plaque builds up on artery walls. Plaque is a sticky, yellow substance made of fatty substances like cholesterol as well as calcium and waste products from your cells. It narrows and clogs the arteries, slowing the flow of blood. This condition is called atherosclerosis, which may begin as early as childhood. It can occur anywhere in the body, but it usually affects large and medium-sized arteries.

Sometimes plaque in an artery can rupture. The body's repair system creates a blood clot to heal the wound. But the clot can block the artery, leading to either a heart attack or a stroke.

The factors that cause plaque to build up are:

- Damage or injury to the inner layer of the coronary arteries caused by the risk factors listed above

- Plaque accumulates at the site of the injury in a process called atherosclerosis, or hardening of the arteries.

Symptoms

Early warning signs may include:

- fatigue

- pain

- dizziness

They can also include the symptoms that are most associated with angina:

- A squeezing, suffocating, or burning feeling in your chest that tends to start in the center of your chest but may move to your arm, neck, back, throat, or jaw

Women are more likely to experience non-traditional symptoms such as:

- vague chest discomfort

- fatigue

- sleep difficulties

- indigestion

- anxiety

If left untreated, CAD can lead to other serious problems such as heart attack, stroke, or even death.

2. Arrhythmia disorder

Usually, a heart beats between 60 and 80 times per minute, but everyone has their own normal heartbeat rhythm. Some hearts beat faster or more slowly than others. When you are diagnosed with arrhythmia, it is an abnormal heart rhythm for you, but not necessarily for someone else.

The pumping action of your heart is triggered by electrical impulses that begin in your heart's natural pacemaker, called the sinus node (also called the sinoatrial or SA node). Learn how a healthy heart works.

Arrhythmia may cause your heart to beat too slowly (bradycardia, less than 60 beats per minute) or too quickly (tachycardia, more than 100 beats per minute) or cause uncoordinated contractions (fibrillation).

Types of arrhythmia

Arrhythmias are defined by the speed of the heartbeats: slow and fast. They include bradycardia and tachycardia, with a variety of conditions falling under those two categories.

1. Slow heart beat—bradycardia

Bradycardia occurs when your heart beats so slowly that it cannot pump enough blood for your body's needs. Untreated bradycardia can cause excessive tiredness, dizziness, lightheadedness, or fainting. An electronic pacemaker can help the heart beat normally.

Bradycardia can be caused by:

- **Sick sinus syndrome**

  This is a malfunction in the heart's natural pacemaker (the sinus node), which makes it fire too slowly. This condition may be caused by growing older or by disease. Some medications can also cause or aggravate a slow heartbeat. The resulting arrhythmia may be temporary or permanent. It can be treated with medication or with an electronic pacemaker.

- **Heart block**

This is the slowing down or interruption of the electrical signal to the lower chambers of the heart, which causes the heart muscle to contract. The heart's electrical system normally sends signals from the upper chambers of the heart (atria) to the lower chambers (ventricles) in a pattern that causes a heartbeat, a coordinated contraction of the heart muscle.

2. Rapid heartbeat(tachycardia)a

Tachycardia occurs when your heart beats too fast. There are two main types: tachycardia above a ventricle and tachycardia in a ventricle.

- **Tachycardia above a ventricle (supraventricular)**
  These are rapid heartbeats in the atria (the top chambers of your heart) or in the AV (atrioventricular) node, the electrical connection between the atria and the ventricles (the lower chambers of your heart).

- **Atrial flutter**
  in atrial flutter, an extra or early electrical impulse travels around and

around the atria in a circular path rather than down along its normal path. This electrical signal causes the atria to "flutter," contracting at a much higher rate than normal. Atrial flutter is usually not life-threatening but can cause chest pain, faintness, or other more serious problems.

- **Atrial fibrillation (Afib)**
  This common form of tachycardia occurs when the electrical activity in the atria is disorganized and very rapid. The pattern of electrical activity stimulates the atria randomly and at a high speed, which causes a series of very rapid contractions of the heart's upper chambers, preventing them from pumping effectively. Though not usually life-threatening, the rapid, irregular, and uncoordinated beating of the ventricles may cause light-headedness or palpitations. If it goes on for several

days or longer, it may increase your risk of stroke because blood trapped in the atria can clot and travel from your heart to your brain, causing a stroke.

- **Paroxysmal supraventricular tachycardia (PSVT)**
This type of tachycardia produces heart rates between 140 and 250 beats per minute. PSVT usually occurs in people who are born with an extra electrical circuit or pathway between the atria and the ventricles. PSVT often starts when you are young, but it may also start later in life. It may be distressing, but it is rarely life-threatening.

- **Wolff-Parkinson-White (WPW) Syndrome**
if you have WPW syndrome, an extra, abnormal electrical pathway in your heart leads to tachycardia. The abnormality is present at birth

(congenital), but WPW is usually diagnosed in adolescence or early adulthood. Most people with WPW syndrome lead normal lives. Many have no symptoms and no episodes of tachycardia. Some people experience rapid heartbeats (paroxysmal supraventricular tachycardia), with heart rates rising up to 240 beats per minute. Other symptoms include palpitations, shortness of breath, fainting, and possibly **angina**.

Tachycardia in a ventricle

- **Ventricular tachycardia**
  Ventricular tachycardia occurs when the ventricles (the lower chambers of the heart) beat too fast. The ventricles are responsible for pumping blood to the rest of the body. If tachycardia becomes so severe that the ventricles can't pump effectively, it may be life-threatening.

Ventricular tachycardia can be treated with medications. Other treatments include an implantable defibrillator, catheter ablation, non-surgical procedures to destroy malfunctioning cells, or surgery to remove damaged heart tissue.

- **Ventricular fibrillation** incorrectly timed electrical signals or signals that do not follow normal pathways may set off ventricular fibrillation. Like atrial fibrillation, the electrical signal that normally triggers a heartbeat splits and goes off on random paths around the ventricles instead of following its normal route. This causes a series of rapid, but ineffective, contractions of the ventricles. Without treatment, ventricular fibrillation may be fatal. Treatment is an electric shock to the heart using a machine called a defibrillator. The shock resets the heart and returns it to its normal rhythm.

- **Postural orthostatic tachycardia syndrome (POTS)**
  POTS makes it difficult to adjust to a standing position from a lying-down position. People with POTS experience a rapid heartbeat that can increase up to 120 beats per minute within 10 minutes of standing. Other common symptoms include headaches, lightheadedness, inability to exercise, extreme fatigue, sweating, nausea, chest discomfort, brain fog (mental clouding), and near fainting (syncope).

POTS commonly appears between the ages of 12 and 50 and typically affects more females than males. To diagnose POTS, your doctor will measure your blood pressure and heart rate while you're lying down and standing up. Measurements are taken immediately after changing positions, as well as at 2, 5, and 10-minute intervals after standing up. POTS is frequently misdiagnosed as panic attacks or chronic anxiety. Sometimes a test called a head upright tilt table exam will be performed to help confirm the diagnosis.

Although POTS can be a severely debilitating disorder, many patients will slowly improve over time, and the majority will respond to treatment.

Causes

Electrical system malfunctions that lead to a heart rhythm disorder can be caused by many things. The list includes:

- damage to the heart from a heart attack

- high blood pressure

- heart valve disease

- congenital heart disease

- cardiomyopathy

- inherited rhythm disorders

- diabetes

- thyroid problems

- alcohol

- caffeine

- smoking

- drugs and supplements

- stress

- sleep apnea

Symptoms

There are many types of arrhythmias; some have no symptoms or warning signs, some are not very serious, and others may be life-threatening.

Symptoms vary from person to person depending on how healthy your heart is, the type of arrhythmia you have, how severe it is, how often it happens, and how long it lasts.

Some arrhythmias do not have any warning signs.

Arrhythmias may decrease the blood flow in your brain and body, causing heart palpitations, dizziness, fainting, or even death. If you have bradycardia, you may feel tired, short of breath, dizzy, or faint. If you have tachycardia, your heartbeat might feel like a strong pulse in your neck or a fluttering, racing beat in your chest. You may also feel discomfort in your chest, weakness, and shortness of breath, faintness, sweatiness, or dizziness. If you have any of these symptoms, see your doctor immediately.

3: structural heart disease

The term "structural heart disease" describes conditions that affect the heart's valves, walls, muscles, or blood vessels close to the heart. It may be congenitally present at birth or acquired after birth as a result of an infection, normal wear and tear, or other circumstances.

Every age and stage of life requires assistance for those with heart problems and their families, who frequently need continuing medical care and surgical operations.

Valvular heart disease

Four chambers make up the heart. The left and right ventricles are the two lower chambers, while the left and right atrium are the two upper chambers. Blood flows continuously in one direction from the heart to the lungs and the rest of the body thanks to the four valves at the exit of each chamber.

The four valves are the tricuspid valve, pulmonary valve, mitral valve, and aortic valve.

- Oxygen-poor blood coming into your heart from your body flows into the right atrium. The tricuspid valve is the valve between the right atrium and the right ventricle. It opens so blood can be pumped to the right ventricle.

- The pulmonary valve controls blood flow between the right ventricle and the lungs. It opens to let the heart pump blood out of the ventricles into the pulmonary artery towards the lungs so it can pick up oxygen. The oxygen-rich blood flows back from the lungs into the left atrium.

- The mitral valve lies between the left atrium and the left ventricle. It opens so the oxygen-rich blood from the left atrium can be pumped into the left ventricle.

- The aortic valve controls blood flow from the left ventricle into the aorta (the main artery in your body). When this valve opens, the oxygen-rich blood is pumped to the aorta and then out to fuel the rest of your body.

In between each step, the valve closes to prevent blood from flowing backwards and mixing oxygen-poor blood with oxygen-rich blood. The one-way, continuous flow of blood delivers oxygen throughout your body.

Heart valve disease occurs when one or more of the heart valves do not open or close properly. When it affects more than one heart valve, it is called multiple valvular heart disease.

- **Stenosis occurs** when the valve opening becomes narrow and restricts blood flow.

- **Prolapse is** when a valve slips out of place or the valve flaps (leaflets) do not close properly.

- **Regurgitation is** when blood leaks backward through a valve, sometimes due to prolapse.

Heart valve disease can be classified as mild, moderate, or severe. It can lead to an enlarged heart or heart failure. Heart failure is a serious medical condition where the heart cannot pump enough blood to meet the body's need for oxygen.

Many valvular heart diseases can be treated with medication, surgery, and other procedures to repair or replace the valve.

Types of valvular heart disease

1. Valvular stenosis (narrowing)

The stiffening of heart valves can narrow the size of the valve opening and restrict blood flow. The narrowing is called valve stenosis. It keeps the valve from opening fully and reduces the amount of blood that can flow through. In severe cases, the valve opening can become so narrow that the rest of the body may not receive adequate blood flow.

- **Tricuspid valve stenosis** if your tricuspid valve narrows, blood is not able to fully move from the right atrium to the right ventricle. This can cause the atrium to enlarge, affecting pressure and blood flow in the surrounding chambers and veins. It can also cause the right ventricle to become smaller, so less blood circulates to your lungs to pick up oxygen.

- **Pulmonary valve stenosis** if your pulmonary valve narrows, the flow of oxygen-poor blood from the right ventricle through the pulmonary arteries to the lungs is restricted. This affects your blood's ability to pick up oxygen and deliver oxygen-rich blood to the rest of your body. With pulmonary valve stenosis, the right ventricle has to work harder to pump blood through the narrowed pulmonary valve, and the pressure in the heart is often increased.

- **Mitral valve stenosis** when the mitral valve narrows, blood flow from the left atrium to the left ventricle is reduced. This can cause fatigue and shortness of breath because the volume of blood carrying oxygen from the lungs is reduced. Pressure from the blood that has stayed in the left atrium can cause the atrium to enlarge and fluid to build up in the lungs.

- **Aortic valve stenosis** When the aortic valve narrows, blood flow from your heart to your aorta (the main artery to your body) and onwards to the rest of your body is restricted. As a result, the left ventricle has to contract harder to try to push blood across the aortic valve. This can often lead to thickening of the left ventricle (left vernacular hypertrophy), which eventually makes the heart less efficient.

2. Valvular prolapse (slipping out of place)

Prolapse is a condition when the valve flaps (leaflets) slip out of place or form a bulge. This can lead to improper or uneven closure of the heart valve. As a result of the prolapsed valve, blood may leak backwards through the valve, and one-way blood flow may be disrupted.

- **Mitral valve prolapse** in mitral valve prolapse, the valve fails to close evenly. Part or all of the mitral valve bulges upward into the atrium when the two ventricles contract. This can allow a small amount of blood to leak backward through the valve (regurgitation). Mitral valve prolapse is also called click-murmur syndrome, Barlow's syndrome, or floppy valve syndrome.

- **Tricuspid, pulmonary, and aortic valve prolapse** these prolapses are less common than mitral valve prolapses. Similar to mitral valve prolapse, the leaflets of the valve do not close completely and fail to form a tight seal.

3. Regurgitation (leaking)

Regurgitation can happen when the valve doesn't close properly and allows blood to flow backwards. This disruption of the one-way blood flow in the heart puts a strain on your heart, reduces its pumping efficiency, and limits its ability to supply your body with oxygen-rich blood.

- **Tricuspid valve regurgitation** when the tricuspid valve does not close properly, blood that is being pumped forward from the right ventricle to the lungs can leak backward into the right atrium, and the atrium may become enlarged.

- **Pulmonary valve regurgitation** this results when the pulmonary valve doesn't close properly. The lower right chamber (right ventricle) of the heart pushes blood through the pulmonary artery into the lungs for blood to pick up oxygen. When the pulmonary valve does not close completely, blood can leak back from the lungs into the heart. This backward blood flow mixes oxygen-poor and oxygen-rich blood and reduces the availability of oxygen-rich blood to fuel the rest of your body.

- **Mitral valve regurgitation** in mitral valve regurgitation, some blood leaks backward into the left atrium through the mitral valve from the lower chamber as it contracts. This reduces the amount of blood that flows to the rest of the body. As a result of regurgitation, the blood volume and pressure are increased in the left atrium. In severe cases, the increase in volume and pressure may lead to enlargement of the atrium and the buildup of fluid (congestion) in the lungs.

- **Aortic valve regurgitation** this results when oxygen-rich blood leaks backward from the aorta into the left ventricle with each heartbeat. Your body does not get enough blood, and the heart has to work harder to make up for it. Over time, the walls of the ventricle may thicken (hypertrophy). This can increase your risk of heart failure.

Causes

Valvular heart disease can develop before or at birth **(congenital causes), or** normal valves may become damaged during one's lifetime (acquired causes). The cause of valvular heart disease is not always known. Support for more research into the causes of valvular heart disease is needed.

1. **Congenital causes**

- **Congenital valvular heart disease** this is a birth defect that may involve a heart valve being the wrong size or shape, or its valve flaps (leaflets) not being properly attached to the heart.

- **Bicuspid aortic valve disease** a congenital defect that affects the aortic valve. Instead of the normal three leaflets, the bicuspid aortic valve has only two leaflets. Without the third leaflet, the valve is unable to open or close properly, is more prone to aortic valve stenosis, and may lead to regurgitation.

- **Marfan syndrome** this is a genetic disorder that affects the body's connective tissue. Connective tissue holds all the body's cells, organs, and tissues together, including the heart. People with Marfan syndrome may develop mitral valve prolapse and aortic valve regurgitation.

2. Acquired causes

- Rheumatic fever_this is an inflammatory disease that can affect the heart valves if it isn't treated properly. Rheumatic fever usually starts with strep throat or an infection involving strep (streptococcal bacteria). Heart valves may be damaged or scarred as the body fights the strep infection.

- Infective (bacterial) endocarditis: common germs can travel through the bloodstream to the heart and infect the surface of the heart, including the heart valves. People with valvular heart disease are at a higher risk of developing infective endocarditis.

- **Radiation therapy** People who had radiation therapy to the chest due to cancer are more likely to develop valvular heart disease.

- **Age-related heart** valve problems may result from degenerative changes or the normal "wear and tear" of ageing.

3. **Other causes**

- coronary artery disease

- damage to the heart muscle from a heart attack

- other diseases of the heart muscle (cardiomyopathy)

- metabolic disorders such as high blood cholesterol

- tumor in the heart

- Certain medications.

Symptoms

Many people do not notice any symptoms until their blood flow has been significantly reduced by valvular heart disease. Symptoms can include:

- **Chest discomfort, pressure, or tightness (angina)** along the front of your body between your neck and upper abdomen

- **Palpitations (irregular** or rapid heartbeats caused by problems with the heart's electrical system) can sometimes be a symptom of valvular heart disease. Your heart may be working harder. That can cause your heart to enlarge and affect normal heart rhythm, leading to arrhythmia.

- **Shortness of breath,** especially when you are active. Valvular heart disease reduces the amount of oxygen available to fuel your body, and that causes breathlessness.

- **Fatigue or weakness.** You may find it harder to do routine activities such as walking or housework.

- **Light-headedness, dizziness, or near fainting are** most common with aortic stenosis.

- **Swelling can** occur when valve problems cause blood to back up in other parts of the body, leading to fluid buildup and a swollen abdomen, feet, and ankles.

If you don't have many symptoms or if they are mild and not affecting you too much, your doctor may choose to monitor your condition carefully and wait until it is necessary to treat your symptoms. It is important to understand that the symptoms of valvular heart disease may not necessarily reflect the seriousness of the problem. Be sure to have regular check-ups and discuss any changes in your health that you notice with your doctor.

Women are more susceptible than men to valvular heart disease caused by rheumatic fever. Women should be especially careful about any strep infection (streptococcal bacteria).

Women with a history of heart disease should consult their doctor if they are planning a pregnancy. Pregnancy is often associated with significant changes in blood flow and blood pressure, which can aggravate valvular heart disease and increase the risk of an adverse cardiac event.

4. Heart failure

Heart failure is a chronic condition caused by the heart not functioning as it should or a problem with its structure. It can happen if the heart is too weak, too stiff, or both. This can lead to fatigue, swelling in the legs and abdomen, and shortness of breath, which can be from fluid in the lungs.

Congestive heart failure

Is on the rise as more people survive heart attacks and other acute heart conditions. As people with damaged hearts live longer, they become more susceptible to heart failure.

Heart failure is a serious condition. There is no cure. However, with lifestyle changes and treatment options, you can manage your condition very well. Many patients can lead a full and normal life. Learning about your heart failure is an important first step in managing your condition.

Causes

Heart failure has many causes or underlying risk factors. The most common are damage to the heart muscle caused by a heart attack (myocardial infarction) and coronary artery disease.

Another common cause of heart failure is high blood pressure (hypertension). If left undiagnosed and untreated for a long period, high blood pressure can lead to heart failure. It is important to get your blood pressure checked at least once every two years or more often if your physician recommends you do so.

Less common causes include:

- heart valves that are not working properly because they are too narrow or leaky (heart valve disease)

- congenital heart disease

- infection causing inflammation of the heart muscle (myocarditis)

- heart muscle disease of unknown causes

- heart rhythm disorders (arrhythmia)

- other medical conditions such as thyroid diseases or anemia

Symptoms

When your heart doesn't pump well and congestion occurs, you may experience some of these symptoms. Contact your doctor or healthcare provider if any of the following occur:

- Increased shortness of breath, especially when lying flat.

- sudden gain of more than 1.5 kg (3 pounds) over 1 to 2 days, or 2.5 kg (5 pounds) in a single week

- bloating or feeling full all the time

- cough or cold symptoms that last for longer than a week

- tiredness, loss of energy, or extreme tiredness

- loss of or change in appetite

- increased swelling of the ankles, feet, legs, sacrum (base of the spine), or abdomen (stomach area)

- increased urination at night

- cool extremities

- new experience of cognitive impairment (confusion and trouble thinking clearly)

By using your heart failure zone chart, you can make it easier to monitor your condition.

5, Cardiomyopathy

(char-dee-o-my-OP-uh-thee) is a disease of the heart muscle that makes it harder for the heart to pump blood to the rest of the body. Cardiomyopathy can lead to heart failure.

The main types of cardiomyopathy include dilated, hypertrophic, and restrictive cardiomyopathy. Treatment—which might include medications, surgically implanted devices, heart surgery, or, in severe cases, a heart transplant—depends on the type of cardiomyopathy and how serious it is.

Type

Dilated cardiomyopathy

Dilated cardiomyopathy causes the chambers of the heart to grow larger. Untreated, dilated cardiomyopathy can lead to heart failure.

Symptoms of dilated cardiomyopathy, such as fatigue and shortness of breath, can mimic other health conditions. A person with dilated cardiomyopathy might not notice any symptoms at first. But dilated cardiomyopathy can become life-threatening. It's a common cause of heart failure.

Dilated cardiomyopathy is more common in men than women. Treatment of dilated cardiomyopathy may include medications or surgery to implant a medical device that controls the heartbeat or helps the heart pump blood. Sometimes, a heart transplant is needed.

Hypertrophic cardiomyopathy (HCM)

Hypertrophic cardiomyopathy (HCM) is a disease in which the heart muscle becomes thickened (hypertrophied). The thickened heart muscle can make it harder for the heart to pump blood.

Hypertrophic cardiomyopathy often goes undiagnosed because many people with the disease have few, if any, symptoms. However, in a small number of people with HCM, the thickened heart muscle can cause shortness of breath, chest pain, or changes in the heart's electrical system, resulting in life-threatening irregular heart rhythms (arrhythmias) or sudden death.

Symptoms

There might be no signs or symptoms in the early stages of cardiomyopathy. But as the condition advances, signs and symptoms usually appear, including:

- Breathlessness with activity or even at rest

- Swelling of the legs, ankles, and feet

- Bloating of the abdomen due to fluid buildup

- Cough while lying down

- Difficulty lying flat to sleep

- Fatigue

- Heartbeats that feel rapid, pounding, or fluttering

- Chest discomfort or pressure

- Dizziness, lightheadedness, and fainting

Signs and symptoms tend to get worse unless treated. In some people, the condition worsens quickly; in others, it might not worsen for a long time.

Chapter 2

Who has a higher risk of developing heart disease?

Age plays a vital role in the deterioration of cardiovascular functionality, resulting in an increased risk of cardiovascular disease (CVD) in older adults. The prevalence of CVD has also been shown to increase with age in both men and women, including the prevalence of atherosclerosis, stroke, and myocardial infarction. The American Heart Association (AHA) reports that the incidence of CVD in US men and women is ~40% from 40–59 years, ~75% from 60–79 years, and ~86% in those above the age of 80. Thus, older adults present a major burden for the current US healthcare infrastructure due to the high prevalence of CVD. The burden of CVD is directly related to increased mortality, morbidity, and frailty in affected individuals, which also translates to significant overall healthcare costs. Given that the aged US population is expected to increase by 2050 by as much as two- and three-fold, the need for a better understanding of the aetiologies associated with CVD in older adults is critically needed.

Many risk factors have been linked to the development of CVD, such as hypertension, diabetes, and obesity. However, sex differences are also frequently observed in ageing adults with regards to both the onset and prevalence of CVD. In the AHA 2019 Heart Disease and Stroke Statistical Update, the incidence of CVD was reported to be 77.2% in males and 78.2% in females, from ages 60–79 years. Furthermore, the incidence of CVD was reported to be 89.3% in males and 91.8% in females in adults over 80 years of age. With respect to coronary artery disease (CAD), the strongest risk factors are male gender and age. Overall, sex differences that lead to discrepancies in CVD risk factors and outcomes between men and women are largely attributed to sex hormones and their associated receptors. Given the wide gap in cardiac risk factors between premenopausal and postmenopausal women, oestrogen (E2) has been studied extensively for its potential cardioprotective activity. However, hormone replacement therapies (HRT) that utilize oestrogen treatment are largely controversial due to the potential for severe side effects. In this review, we discuss the current understanding of the impact of age on the development and incidence of CVD, with a particular focus on gender discrepancies in CVD in aged adults, in order to provide a better understanding of the considerations needed in the development of future treatments within the ageing population.

Functional changes in ageing adult's hearts have been characterized, which include reports of diastolic and systolic dysfunction and also electrical dysfunction, including the development of arrhythmias. Collectively, both functional and electrical defects result in a high prevalence of heart failure, atrial fibrillation, and other CVDs in ageing patients. The high prevalence of CVD in this population has been linked to a number of factors, including increased oxidative stress, inflammation, apoptosis, overall myocardial deterioration, and degeneration. An increase in the production of reactive oxygen species (ROS) is known to occur with the onset of advanced age and is linked to persistent inflammation and progression to chronic disease status, as in CVD. Increased production of proinflammatory markers is a hallmark of aged hearts, including high levels of interleukin-6 (IL-6), tumor necrosis factor-α (TNF), and CRP (C-reactive protein). Production of inflammatory factors and other mediators contributes to cardiac remodeling, including significant extracellular matrix

(ECM) remodeling, which is caused by impaired ECM turnover. Dysregulation in matrix metalloproteinase (MMP) and tissue inhibitor of metalloproteinase (TIMP) expression levels is frequently linked to increased collagen deposition and the development of cardiac hypertrophy and fibrosis in aged hearts. Fibrosis and hypertrophy are both significant structural changes that lead to eventual cardiac dysfunction in ageing patients. Fibrosis, due to impaired ECM turnover, has been shown to develop in the atria of ageing patients, which also results in atrial fibrillation in many of these patients.

Oxidative stress, including the production of excess ROS that occurs with cardiac ageing, will also lead to mitochondrial function. Cardiac aerobic metabolism is greatly dependent on mitochondrial production of ATP; thus, the loss of mitochondrial function plays a major role in the development of cardiac dysfunction in ageing adults. It has been reported that mitochondrial DNA is particularly susceptible to oxidative damage since it lacks protective histones and is in close proximity to ROS production during electron transport. ROS production has also been shown to impair the efficiency of mitochondrial respiration, which also contributes to the cardiac ageing process via augmented ROS production. Mitochondrial oxidative stress has also been shown to result in impaired calcium signaling via dysregulation of the type 2 ryanodine receptor (RyR2). RyR2, a calcium ion channel, is primarily responsible for the release of calcium from the sarcoplasmic reticulum, allowing for muscle contraction. Decreased activity of the sarcoplasmic reticulum Ca^{2+} ATPase pump (SERCA) has also been observed with age. The generation of biologically active lipid mediators may also result in a response to age-related inflammation. Mitochondrial dysfunction due to increased ROS has been reported to result in the production of lipid oxidation, which has been linked to the development of atherosclerosis. Although impaired lipid metabolism via mitochondrial dysfunction is known to occur with age, this process is still not completely understood. One experimental study in mice reported that diets enriched with omega-6 in older mice lead to chronic low-grade inflammation and impaired oxidative-redox balance, resulting in electrocardiographic disturbances. Collectively, age-related oxidative stress results in significant cellular and structural changes, and these eventually lead to impaired cardiac functionality and the development of CVD.

Prevalence of Cardiovascular Diseases in Ageing and Elderly Adults

Age is a significant independent risk factor for CVD since it is associated with an increased likelihood of the development of any number of other additional cardiac risk factors, including obesity and diabetes. The prevalence of most types of CVD is considerably higher among older adults as compared with the general population. According to the AHA, between the years 2013–2017, 77.8% of women and 70.8% of males in the range of 65–74 years were diagnosed with high blood pressure, or hypertension. Rates of diagnosed hypertension increased drastically to 85.6% in women and 80.0% in men aged over 75 years. Hypertension is a major risk factor for CVD, and it has been linked to several factors such as alcohol consumption, nutrition, smoking, and obesity. Among older adults, hypertension is particularly associated with age, female gender, and obesity. According to the AHA, coronary heart disease (CHD) is more common in older men than in older women. Heart failure with preserved ejection fraction (HF and EF) is more common in the elderly and is more common in older women than in older men. Regarding myocardial infarction (MI) in adults aged 60–79 years, 11.5% of men had a diagnosed MI, while only 4.2% of women were diagnosed with MI. Rates of diagnosed MI are also higher in men over 80 years of age as compared with women. However, this data does not reflect the potential discrepancies related to the diagnosis of acute coronary syndrome in women, including reported underdiagnoses and misdiagnosis of cardiac events in women, including MI.

Arrhythmias are also found to increase with age and are reported to be one of the major risk factors for sudden cardiac death. Among elderly adults aged 66 to 93 years old, persistent atrial fibrillation (AF) was reported in approximately 10% of the outpatient population above the age of 66 years. AF generated about 1.5% of strokes in adults aged 50–59 years and up to 23.5% of strokes in older adults aged 80–89 years. According to the AHA, in those hospitalized for stroke from ages 65 to 84 years, females and males had approximately equal inpatient hospital stays, but women ≥85 years accounted for nearly 66% of all stroke patients. With the number of incident strokes projected to increase twofold over the next 40 years (2010–2050), the geriatric population (≥75 years old) is likely to experience the bulk of these potentially fatal events.

The Prevalence of Ageing Adults Admitted to Critical Care

Risks associated with age present an inimitable difficulty with regards to medical treatment, especially with respect to critical and intensive care treatments. Given that the prevalence of health complications increases with advanced age, it is no surprise that the average age of patients admitted to the ICU is approximately 60 years. However, advanced age has been reported to be associated with increased mortality in ICU patients, even after controlling for preexisting morbidities. Thus, advanced age is a risk for mortality in ICU patients. Regardless of treatment intensity. While age is an independent risk factor for mortality in ICU patients, the presence of health conditions and diseases is known to significantly augment the risk of mortality in these patients. Thus, a higher prevalence of CVD in elderly ICU patients has been reported, including higher rates of heart failure, arrhythmia, and valvular heart disease. High mortality rates due to CVD in critically ill patients have even resulted in the implementation of specialized health units for cardiac patients, referred to as coronary care units (CCU), or more recently, cardiovascular intensive care units (CICU).

Another risk for ageing adult ICU patients is the use of mechanical ventilation. The average age of ventilated patients in the ICU is ~60 years. Importantly, both age and length of ventilation are associated with mortality in ICU patients. Advanced age is also an important factor associated with an increased risk of failed extubation. Studies demonstrate that approximately 35% of elderly patients are reintubated within 48 to 72 hours after extubation. Ventilation with high levels of supplemental oxygen presents another potential risk for elderly patients. Supplemental oxygen is frequently implemented for the treatment of hypoxia in order to improve arterial oxygen levels in critically ill patients. However, high oxygen exposure (hyperoxia) has also been shown to induce oxidative stress due to increased production of ROS, which results in significant lung injury. Additionally, hyperoxia is known to induce hemodynamic changes, including the appearance of decreased heart rate, stroke volume, and cardiac output in patients. Of critical concern, hyperoxia in critically ill patients is also strongly associated with increased risks for poor outcomes and high mortality rates.

Reports suggest that cardiac patients may be at a greater risk for worsened outcomes with supplemental oxygen exposure. One study reported that hyperoxia in MI patients is associated with increased infarct size, recurrent MI, and the development of arrhythmias. The cardiac impact of hyperoxia exposure in patients has not been well defined, but there are certain experimental reports in animal models that suggest a significant cardiac risk. Experimental reports of hyperoxia exposure have demonstrated negative cardiac effects in rabbits, rats, and mice. In mice, the effects of high levels of supplemental oxygen have shown disparate effects in females, including higher rates of mortality and more severe repolarization defects. These results suggest that special therapeutic considerations are needed for ventilation in patients with advanced age, sex, and CVD upon admission to the ICU.

Management and Treatment of CVD in Older Adults

While age is shown to be independently associated with inflammation and a risk for CVD, health behaviors may also complicate these factors. Health behaviors that are commonly linked with poor outcomes in CVD patients include inactivity, poor nutrition, and smoking. The AHA reported that these health behaviors, in addition to poor sleep behavior, are all associated with a higher risk of developing CVD. Self-management of these health behaviors, under the direction of medical care specialists, has shown promise in CVD patients. Thus, lifestyle modifications are a key to promoting better health in ageing adults and are a fundamental approach to reducing cardiovascular risk in adults. Examples of lifestyle changes that have been directly linked to decreased risk of CVD include maintenance of a healthy weight, avoidance of tobacco products, and regular exercise. Diet supplementation with inorganic nitrate has demonstrated beneficial effects on vascular function in older adults via improvements in endothelial function. Thus, inorganic nitrates may also reduce vascular stiffness and thus the risk of atherosclerosis. Enhanced endothelial function and vascular flexibility following mineral nitrate supplementation have been shown to lead to an overall reduction in systolic pressure, particularly in older adults with mild hypertension. Endothelial function may also be improved by the addition of dietary antioxidants. Vitamin C, vitamin E, polyphenols, and carotenoids have all been shown to reduce oxidative stress and thereby may provide a protective effect against CVD. Antioxidants are reported to work primarily by reducing the production of ROS, typically associated with advancing age, which may help to avoid the initiation of the inflammatory cascade. Excess ROS results in the oxidation of lipoprotein (LDL), which is also shown to result in the development of CVD. Reduction of ROS by antioxidants prevents the uptake of oxidized LDL into macrophages, avoiding their conversion into foam cells, and further prevents these from adhering to the endothelium, which would otherwise result in the development of atherosclerotic lesions. The use of antioxidants has also been shown to prevent the release of destructive inflammatory cytokines, which play a crucial role in the activation of the inflammatory cascade.

Physical inactivity has been reported to be a major cause of chronic illnesses, such as

CVD. Regarding the benefit of physical activity, walking has been reported to aid older men in the management of coronary heart disease. Additionally, regular walking activity may increase longevity by decreasing the risk of CVD and other age-related diseases. Additionally, exercise has been shown to be particularly beneficial to ageing adults by protecting against age-related adverse systemic and cellular effects of ageing and by reducing cellular senescence. Additionally, exercise is reported to improve endothelial function in older adults, but with certain differences in males and females. Specifically, endurance exercises are more consistently associated with improved endothelial function in males than in postmenopausal women, due to their lack of oestrogen and subsequently increased oxidative stress. Telemedicine and tele monitoring have also gained exposure for their potential to prevent and/or gauge risk factors associated with CVD. Studies show that self-management via mobile and telehealth technologies can improve outcomes in patients with hypertension, such as through the use of mobile blood pressure monitoring. Unfortunately, elderly adults show low participation in these technologies.

In addition to lifestyle changes, statins, a class of lipid-lowering drugs, are typically implemented as a primary measure to prevent CVD. Statins have been reported to reduce total cholesterol in older adults. Statin use has been shown to result in a 31% decrease in low-density lipoprotein (LDL) cholesterol and a 14% increase in high-density lipoprotein (HDL) cholesterol in older adult patients. Statins are associated with decreased all-cause mortality and cardiovascular events in older individuals without an established CVD diagnosis. Overall, statins lower the risk of MI and stroke in older adults. Administration of statins to older adults with diagnosed CVD is reported to result in a 14% decrease in triglyceride levels. Moreover, in one study, statins were found to decrease the risk of MI by 39.4% in older adults as compared with those treated with a placebo. Furthermore, statin treatment has also led to a 23.8% decreased risk of stroke as compared with a placebo. Although statins are the primary medications for atherosclerosis patients, this class of medications is responsible for muscular dysfunction, myopathy, rhabdomyolysis, and elevated creatinine kinase levels. Thus, the risks of this medication for older adults must be carefully examined when considering its overall benefit. Additionally, while statins have been reported to reduce cardiac mortality in patients after MI, one study reported lower rates of reduction for women as compared with men. However, a recent study published findings that demonstrate that women are less likely to participate in recommended statin therapy after their first MI as compared with men, which may partially account for the diminished mortality reduction for women after MI.

Risk Factors Associated with Cardiovascular Diseases among the Elderly

In this review, we explore age as a prominent risk factor in the development of CVD. We have discussed physiological ageing of the heart as a major causative factor in the onset and manifestation of CVD in ageing adults as a result of increased oxidative stress and Flammarion. However, the risk of developing CVD is associated with many factors and is not simply a consequence of aging. Among the factors that are associated with a higher risk of developing CVD is the higher prevalence of co-morbid risk factors in these patients, including frailty, obesity, and diabetes.

Diabetes in the Elderly Population

Diabetes is a major predisposing factor for the development of CVD in the ageing population. Additionally, older diabetics are reported to be at an excessively higher risk for vascular complications due to their potentially longer disease duration. Currently, diabetic cardiomyopathy (DCM) is the primary cause of mortality in diabetic patients. The prevalence of diabetes is very high among adults aged 65 years and over. In older patients and in the general population, type 2 diabetes is the most prevalent. Specifically, among older adults aged 65 years and older, the combined prevalence of diagnosed and undiagnosed prediabetes and diabetes is between 50 and 80%. It has also been projected that the number of patients 65 years of age and older with diagnosed diabetes will increase up to fourfold by 2050.

DCM describes a heart disease that develops in patients primarily due to diabetes. Studies demonstrate that cardiovascular complications, like stroke, ischemia, and angina, are very common in geriatric diabetic patients. While heart disease is the leading cause of mortality in diabetes, and diabetics have a higher risk for mortality due to CVD as compared with nondiabetics, it has been reported that many elderly diabetic patients may be unaware that they have heart disease. Additionally, one study also reported that silent ischemic events may also be more common in elderly diabetics.

Type 2 diabetes mellitus (T2DM) is known to have a gender bias. While the prevalence of T2DM is higher in men, the most prominent risk factor, obesity, is more common in women. Furthermore, cardiovascular risks associated with diabetes also appear to be higher in women. Diabetic women are at a higher risk for heart failure as compared with men, including a higher risk for mortality due to coronary heart disease (CHD). Additionally, mortality due to diabetic cardiomyopathy is also reported to be higher in women than in men. Diabetes also appears to attenuate the protective effect of oestrogen against cardiac disease in premenopausal females. The cardiac disadvantage in diabetic women has been linked to lower levels of high-density lipoprotein cholesterol (HDLC) in these patients as compared with both non-diabetic women and diabetic men.

The risks for the development of type 2 diabetes in older adults are attributed to genetics, lifestyle, and other physiological aspects of ageing, such as inflammation and oxidative stress. These effects, in combination, can cause hyperglycemia through impaired insulin production or insulin sensitivity. In ageing diabetics, poor glucose homeostasis has been shown to be more closely associated with impaired insulin secretion by beta cells than with tissue insulin sensitivity. Additionally, age-related beta cell function has also been linked with certain genetic alterations. Inflammation and inflammatory cytokines also play a key role in the development of type 2 diabetes. Additionally, certain inflammatory markers have been shown to predict mortality due to cardiovascular disease in diabetic patients. In one study, type 2 diabetics with the highest C-reactive protein (CRP) levels were shown to have a 76% greater risk for mortality related to cardiovascular complications. Given that ageing and diabetes are both risk factors for vascular inflammation, a higher risk for CVD is observed in ageing diabetics.

Among adults aged 65 years and older, the risk of developing CVD has also been linked to fetuin-A, a hepatic secretory protein that is synthesized in the liver and secreted into blood serum. Higher concentrations of fetuin-A influence the onset of CVD through increased risk of type 2 diabetes, higher body mass index (BMI), higher waist circumference, higher LDL cholesterol, as well as elevated triglycerides, cholesterol, homeostatic model assessment-insulin resistance (HOMA-IR), and C-reactive protein (CRP) levels. The relationship between fetuin-A and the occurrence of CVD differs between individuals with and without type 2 diabetes. Those with high fetuin-A levels and type 2 diabetes have an 18% higher risk of developing CVD as compared with their non-diabetic counterparts. Overall, there is an inverse association between fetuin-A and CVD in people without type 2 diabetes.

Obesity in the Elderly Population

Age is a major risk factor for CVD, since it represents an increased likelihood of the development of other additional risk factors, including obesity. Obesity, as in diabetes, has been linked to persistent inflammation and oxidative stress .The cardiovascular risks involved with obesity are partially mediated by concurrent presentation of high blood pressure, cholesterol, and glucose. However, one study in patients with high BMI found that interventions which control hypertension, hyperglycemia, and high cholesterol may only reduce the risks for coronary heart disease by half and the risk for stroke by about three-quarters. These results indicate that BMI is an independent risk factor for CVD, which has also been supported by additional studies. Recently, studies have found that centralized adiposity, marked by waist circumference and/or waist-to-height ratio, is a better indicator of CVD risk factors, including the risk of mortality due to CVD. One study showed that abdominal obesity in the elderly is strongly associated with the prevalence of atherosclerotic cardiovascular disease (ASCVD). Another study indicated that a high waist-to-height ratio in elderly adults is strongly associated with a high cardiovascular risk. Given the prevalence of obesity in adults, as high as 37.5% in men and 39.4% in women over the age of 60, High BMI and/or central adiposity present a significant risk for CVD in the ageing population; the data are also reflective of the higher prevalence of obesity in women than in men. The accumulation of visceral fat in women after menopause has been linked to hormonal changes, such as decreased oestrogen, which result in an increased risk of metabolic syndrome and cardiovascular complications in obese postmenopausal women. Further studies indicate that the risk of BMI-associated CVD mortality is also higher in women than in men. Of critical concern, the prevalence of obesity in older adults is expected to continue to increase.

Frailty in the Elderly Population

Another important risk factor associated with the development and manifestation of CVD among the elderly is the onset of frailty.

Among men and women aged 65 years and over, the presence of significant frailty has been shown to accurately predict incident CVD. Frailty is known to be a direct consequence of a weakened physiological reserve, which results in a heightened vulnerability to either acute or chronic illness. More than 20 frailty measures have been developed, and most of these are used to assess the key phenotypic aspects of frailty, such as decreased walking speed, exhaustion, inactivity, muscle wasting, and weakness. Muscle wasting is commonly associated with frailty in older adults and includes the development of sarcopenia, or significant loss of muscle mass. Studies have shown that the onset of frailty is also strongly associated with a higher incidence of disability, hospital admissions, poor outcomes, and mortality. In a similar way to age-related obesity and diabetes, increased oxidative stress is a risk factor for the onset of frailty in older adults.

Frailty and associated sarcopenia are common outcomes of age-related inflammation and are also augmented in those with metabolic syndrome, including insulin resistance. The frailty phenotype increases the risk of developing CVD through its positive and significant correlation with central adiposity and inflammation, which are both observed at a high prevalence in ageing adults. Sex has also been shown to play a role in the development of frailty in older adults. Females are more likely than men to develop frailty. This may be due, at least in part, to lower baseline muscle mass in women as compared with men. Additionally, one study reported that frailty in females may also be a stronger independent predictor of mortality than in males.

Sex Differences That Arise from Hormones in Ageing Adults

Within the context of this review, we have discussed several differences in CVD risk factors that are associated with sex in ageing adults. While age is an independent risk factor for CVD in both men and women, it is evident that older women are more prone to certain complications that are related to heart disease. Generally, before menopause, women are relatively protected from cardiovascular disease, and then, after menopause, the risk for cardiac disease greatly increases in women. The decline of sex hormones has been shown to play an important role in the development of CVD with the onset of advanced age in both men and women. Thus, we discuss the roles of both oestrogen and testosterone in CVD in older adults.

The Impact of Oestrogen on CVD in Ageing Adults

Oestrogen is often recognized for its cardioprotective role and is reported to be directly associated with the overall lower incidence of CVD in premenopausal women as compared with age-matched men. Oestrogen has been shown to exert a cardioprotective effect in males as well. One study reported that males are likely to develop heart disease 10–15 years earlier than women due to the gradual decline in oestrogen levels after puberty. Conversely, men of 70 years of age have lower overall cardiovascular risk as compared with women at age 50, the average age of menopause in women. Which is a strong indication that oestrogen decline has a greater impact on CVD risks in women than in men. It has been reported that the risk for CVD increases dramatically in women at the onset of menopause, by as much as 2–4 times. In addition to increased risk for CVD, women at menopause are also at a greater risk for high

LDL cholesterol levels, hypertension, diabetes, and obesity, which further elevates cardiovascular risk factors in both premenopausal and postmenopausal women. Clinical studies report a high incidence of CAD in young women who have undergone bilateral oophorectomy, providing further support for the likely cardioprotective role of oestrogen since the most abundant form of oestrogen, 17-beta-estradiol, is secreted primarily by the ovaries. Experimental studies in mice have also reported the cardioprotective effect in both males and females via mechanisms that include those that support mitochondrial homeostasis and reduce oxidative stress. Other experimental studies in mice have supported the effects of oestrogen and include mechanisms that promote neo-angiogenesis and those that prevent fibrosis.

Because of the heightened cardiovascular risks in women after menopause, oestrogen replacement therapy has been studied as a potential therapy for CVD. However, to date, the effects of oestrogen replacement on cardiovascular health are still largely controversial. The Nurse's Health Study published epidemiology data from ~28,000 postmenopausal women with no history of CVD and demonstrated that oestrogen therapy was associated with reductions in CVD incidence and mortality by 40% and 50%, respectively. However, a 20-year follow-up study in this population demonstrated that oestrogen therapy was correlated with an elevated risk for stroke. Further controlled trials have shown that oestrogen replacement therapy is largely associated with increased cardiovascular risks in older women (>67 years) with diagnosed VD. Furthermore, the Heart and Oestrogen/Progestin Replacement Study (HERS) was stopped after only four years due to an increased incidence of MI and death in women undergoing hormone replacement, which was presumed to be due to the higher risks associated with CVD in the older female population. More recent research suggests that oestrogen therapy in women after the onset of menopause may also be the cause of many of the clinical trials involving hormone replacement. There have been reported cardioprotective benefits in women when oestrogen replacement is introduced in early menopause, More study is needed in order to determine if this critical window therapy may also reduce cardiovascular risk for women at an older age.

The Impact of Testosterone on CVD in Ageing Adults

Testosterone, the major sex hormone for men, is also demonstrated to exert cardioprotective function. In men, low testosterone levels due to hypogonadism are correlated with advanced age and other factors, such as obesity. Epidemiological studies report an increased risk for cardiovascular disease in ageing adult men that is associated with hypogonadism, including reduced levels of testosterone. Low testosterone was also shown to be independently associated with a high risk for acute MI in type 2 diabetic males and a high incidence of coronary artery disease (CAD) in men. In older men, low testosterone levels have been linked to a higher risk of stroke. An additional study reported that men, at 40 years of age, who had serum testosterone levels below the recommended threshold level also had a higher mortality risk due to CVD. Since testosterone levels show a decline in both men and women with advanced age, the impact of testosterone on postmenopausal women has also been studied. Subsequently, it was found in one study that low levels of testosterone were also associated with coronary artery disease (CAD) in postmenopausal women.

Epidemiological studies, which have demonstrated a link between low testosterone levels and an increased risk for cardiovascular events, have led to studies involving testosterone replacement as a potential therapy. However, the benefits of testosterone therapy for hormone-deficient men with or without pre-existing cardiovascular disease are largely controversial. One clinical trial reported an increased risk for MI, stroke, and mortality with testosterone therapy, while another trial suggested that testosterone protected men against all of these same risks. In a larger meta-analysis study that reported results from approximately 3000 older men, it was found that men treated with testosterone had a 54% increase in cardiovascular events as compared with those treated with a placebo. In a larger retrospective study with results from 56,000 individuals, it was demonstrated that testosterone therapy in men is linked to a 36% higher risk of MI within three treatments. As of 2019, the US Endocrine Society (ES) reported that there is not sufficient current evidence to accurately assess the cardiovascular effect of testosterone replacement therapy. Thus, the ES recommends caution when implementing testosterone therapy in older men with CVD and further recommends against the use of testosterone replacement in men who have had a cardiovascular event within 6 months. Currently, the ES primarily recommends testosterone therapy for the treatment of pathological hypogonadism in men, such as in disorders involving the hypothalamus, pituitary, and testes. While a majority of men show diminished testosterone levels with advanced age, these levels are still considered within the normal physiological range, without symptoms of androgen deficiency or hypogonadism. However, a small proportion of older men (1–2%) will show evidence of androgen deficiency, including testicular dysfunction and various sexual and physical symptoms. Testosterone therapy for 12 months in this population of older men has demonstrated benefits in sexual function and mood and in certain aspects of vitality, such as increased walking distance. Testosterone was also found to increase hemoglobin levels. It is important to note that these studies did not report major cardioprotective benefits in men with testosterone therapy, and similarly, they did not report any major adverse effects in the heart. Despite the potential benefits of hormone replacement therapy in older men, the US Endocrine Society does not currently recommend testosterone therapy in asymptomatic older men (>65 years), particularly as an "anti-ageing" treatment, due to the lack of complete evidence for the potential long-term risks of hormone therapies, as in potential cardiovascular risks. Cardiovascular disease (CVD) is a major health concern in the ageing population. While age is an independent risk factor for CVD, other additional risk factors that are closely associated with advanced age have been shown to compound these risks, including frailty, obesity, and diabetes. Overall, although females have a longer life expectancy than males, women make up the most significant percentage of CVD diagnoses in the elderly population, or in those greater than 80 years old. These comorbid risks, in combination, are shown to compound cardiovascular risk factors in older patients upon admission to the ICU. Gender is yet another major risk factor regarding the onset, manifestation, and management of CVD in ageing adults. The decline in hormone levels may play a significant role in the development of CVD in older men and women, but hormone replacement therapies have not yet shown a significant benefit in older adults with respect to cardiovascular health. Given that the number of older patients will continue to increase, it is critically necessary to uncover the impact of hormones on cardiovascular risk factors in future clinical and research studies in order to improve outcomes in the older population.

Chapter 3

Unexpected Things That Make Your Heart Hurt

Millions of Americans live with some form of heart disease. This condition is a leading cause of death in the United States. While it's not totally preventable, as age and family history can play a role, there are some things you may be doing right now that are putting you at risk of getting heart disease.

Check out these nine common habits that are bad for your heart.

1. Smoking

Most people know smoking is bad for their lungs. But it's just as bad for your heart. It harms your heart by damaging your blood vessels and raising your blood pressure. It also keeps your body from getting enough oxygen into your blood. Even being around other people while they smoke can cause damage.

2. Drinking too much

There are many links between alcohol and heart disease. Your favorite alcoholic drink might be more harmful than you think. Americans lose their lives every year due to alcohol abuse, alcohol-related accidents, and the effects of long-term drinking. Drinking alcohol can also be harmful for your heart. Here's how.

How alcohol hurts the heart

Alcohol use increases heart attack risk by 40 percent, according to Alcohol.org. This is because drinking often can damage your heart muscle and raise your blood pressure. Some drinks also have high calorie counts. Consuming more calories than your body needs opens the door to problems like obesity. Obesity also increases the risk of developing heart disease.

Dangers of binge drinking

If you have four or five drinks in roughly two hours, you're crossing the line from drinking to binge drinking. Drinking alcohol that fast comes with a unique set of risks. Binge drinking can change your heart's rhythm, which is called arrhythmia. People who have it may notice chest pain or discomfort.

Having six or more servings of hard liquor in a night raises your risk of having a stroke or heart attack too. In fact, the odds of having a stroke or heart attack remain higher for an entire week after binge drinking.

Who should avoid alcohol?

Everyone should do their best to limit their alcohol intake.

If you have a history of heart failure or stroke, high blood pressure, or uneven heartbeats, it can be helpful to avoid alcohol. Ask your doctor about what kind of limits you should stick to.

People with diabetes should also talk to their doctors about their drinking habits. Alcohol can lower your blood sugar levels. If you have diabetes, it's better to enjoy your drink with food. You should also monitor your blood sugar before and after drinking.

Pregnant women and people with a history of alcohol abuse should avoid drinking together. If you drink while taking certain medications, you could also put yourself at risk for issues like nausea, dizziness, and even fainting. In most cases, medicine comes with a label that warns you about the harmful effects that can happen when mixing it with alcohol.

3. **Not getting enough sleep**

Just like the rest of your body, your heart needs rest. After a long or stressful day, your heart rate and blood pressure drop when you fall asleep. This gives your heart the rest it needs. The more restful sleep you get, the better your cardiovascular health can be. Being sleep deprived also stresses your body out, which is another habit that's bad for your heart.

4. **Staying stressed out**

Stressed? Here's the secret to inner peace:

How do I find inner peace even when the world around me feels chaotic?

With the change of seasons often comes the desire to have greater inner peace.

When striving for inner peace, the first step is to understand what inner peace truly is.

Inner peace exists regardless of external conditions. It comes from faith and resilience, and from accepting circumstances the way they are. It also comes from uncluttering our lives with possessions and all the activities that create more burden than joy.

Here are a few tips to help you develop inner peace:

- Breathe deeply, stretch often, eat well, and get enough sleep.

- Give yourself total quiet every day, even for just a few minutes.

- Spend a few of those quiet moments in the presence of your God.

- Face problems instead of trying to escape or deny them.

- Solve the problems you can and accept those you can't.

You're on the way towards inner peace when you find yourself...

- Allowing things to unfold, rather than resisting or controlling them,

- No longer judge others or yourself.

- Disinterested in conflict.

- Feeling the beauty of being alive and enjoying small moments.

- Experiencing a deep connection to others and with nature.

- Focusing on giving and loving rather than receiving.

While many people assume that inner peace will simply arrive some day when everything is right, experts say that it is much more of a conscious effort. Start by taking small steps. This might mean placing a sticky note on your desk reminding you to take deep breaths or writing a grocery list at the beginning of each week that is full of healthy, whole foods.

5. Beginning TV shows

You probably love sitting around and streaming your favorite shows. Who doesn't? Unfortunately, sitting for long periods of time is bad for your heart and can affect the amount of sugar and fat in your blood. Instead of sitting through each episode, watch while you're on the treadmill or exercising. Or, do exercises on your living room floor.

6. Skipping flossing your teeth

Your oral health plays a big role in whether or not you might develop heart disease, especially if you have gum disease. One way to treat or prevent gum disease is to floss your teeth. It's a step many people skip when taking care of their teeth. Many dentists recommend flossing at least twice a day.

7. Eating a poor diet

The 10 Worst Foods for Your Heart

Want to keep heart disease at bay? You might need to make some lifestyle changes. One of the most important is changing the way you eat, particularly if these 10 foods are part of your regular diet. Each one may increase your risk for heart disease, which can lead to a heart attack.

.Candy

It's no secret that candy isn't a healthy food option, but scientists have discovered it might be worse than you might think. Research shows that eating too much sugar can lead to conditions that can cause heart disease, such as high cholesterol, diabetes, obesity, and inflammation.

.Sugary cereals

Sugary cereal is one food that many people have for breakfast each day without realizing how harmful it can be. Eating certain types of cereal every morning can raise your blood sugar and increase the amount of inflammation in your body. These conditions can be harmful to your heart.

.Soda

Those who drink soda frequently are more likely to be obese, have diabetes, and have high blood pressure. And don't assume diet soda is better. While the science isn't settled, diet sodas may increase your risk of gaining weight or having a stroke.

.Alcohol

There are many links between alcohol and heart disease. Your favorite alcoholic drink might be more harmful than you think. Americans lose their lives every year due to alcohol abuse, alcohol-related accidents, and the effects of long-term drinking. Drinking alcohol can also be harmful for your heart. Here's how.

How alcohol hurts the heart

Alcohol use increases heart attack risk by 40 percent, according to Alcohol.org. This is because drinking often can damage your heart muscle and raise your blood pressure. Some drinks also have high calorie counts. Consuming more calories than your body needs opens the door to problems like obesity. Obesity also increases the risk of developing heart disease.

High blood pressure is often called the silent killer due to the millions that have it but are unaware they do. In addition to these millions, one in three adults has been diagnosed with the disease. Whether you've been diagnosed or not, learning how to prevent and control high blood pressure is crucial to your health.

What is high blood pressure?

Blood pressure is measured using two numbers. The first, systolic blood pressure, measures the pressure in your blood vessels when your heart beats. The second, diastolic blood pressure, measures the pressure in your blood vessels when your heart rests between beats.

Without treatment, high blood pressure, also called hypertension, can damage the heart, brain, kidneys, and eyes, which may lead to serious problems such as heart disease, stroke, and kidney failure. Fortunately, it is easy to detect and bring under control.

What causes high blood pressure?

No one knows the exact cause of the condition, but many factors are known to raise blood pressure, including:

- Being overweight or obese

- Consuming an excess of alcohol

- Having a family history of high blood pressure

- Eating a diet high in sodium

- Smoking

- Getting older

How is it detected?

Your primary care doctor would typically diagnose hypertension after readings of 140/90 or higher on three or more separate occasions (usually measured within a week or two).

How is it treated?

Because no one is the same, there isn't just one way to treat high blood pressure. Your health and family history, blood pressure status, and other health conditions are all considered when finding your best treatment options.

How is it prevented?

You can prevent or delay high blood pressure by:

- Staying at a healthy weight or losing extra weight

- Eating less salt and salty foods

- Exercising regularly

- Quitting smoking

- Drinking alcohol in moderation

- Eating a diet rich in fruits, veggies, and low-fat dairy products

.Processed meat

Hot dogs, cold cuts, pepperoni, and sausages—these processed meats may be tasty, but they may also put you at risk for heart problems in the future. Not only are they loaded with sodium, which can lead to high blood pressure, but they are also high in compounds called nitrates. Foods with nitrates can make your blood vessels stiff, so they aren't able to pump blood as well.

.White bread

When it comes to bread, stay away from anything made from refined white flour. The same goes for white grains, like rice and pasta. When your body digests these foods, it stores and uses them much like sugar for energy. This puts you at risk for weight gain, inflammation, and type 2 diabetes.

.Pizza

With processed meat and white bread in the ingredients, you can probably guess why pizza is bad for your heart. It is also high in sodium and can lead to weight gain. When you do indulge, try veggies instead of processed meats for toppings.

.French fries

French fries are loaded with sodium and saturated fat—two things that may put you at risk for heart disease.

Put a healthy twist on French fries with these alternative recipes!

Traditionally, this favorite side is fried in vegetable oil, which adds additional fat and calories. Baking instead of frying helps minimize the amount of oil in your food. Using olive oil is also a better option when it comes to nutrients and minimal processing of the oil.

Instead of using regular potatoes as your French fry base, consider healthier veggies like sweet potatoes or green beans. Even a fruit like avocado tastes great and is a more wholesome option.

Recipe 1: Sweet Potato Fries

Ingredients

2 sweet potatoes, peeled and cut into wedges

3 tablespoons of olive oil

½ teaspoon salt

½ teaspoon pepper

¼ teaspoon paprika

¼ teaspoon garlic powder

Preheat the oven to 425 degrees and spray a baking sheet with cooking spray. Place the sweet potatoes and oil in a large bowl and toss. Sprinkle with salt, pepper, and paprika. Arrange potatoes on a baking sheet evenly and cook for 18 to 24 minutes, flipping occasionally, until golden brown. Cool for 5 minutes before serving.

Recipe 2: Baked French Fries

Ingredients

3 lbs. potatoes

3 tablespoons of olive oil

1 teaspoon salt

1/2 teaspoon pepper

Preheat the oven to 450 degrees and cut the potatoes into fry shapes. Toss potatoes with a mixture of olive oil, salt, and pepper. Bake at 450 degrees for 35 to 40 minutes, flipping once, until golden brown.

Recipe 3: Avocado Fries

Ingredients

3 avocados

3 whisked eggs

1 cup of flour

1 cup panko breadcrumbs

1 teaspoon salt

½ teaspoon cayenne pepper (or substitute with garlic powder)

Slice avocados in half and then lengthwise into wedges. Mix breadcrumbs with cayenne pepper and salt. Roll avocado slices in flour, then eggs, then breadcrumb mixture. Place on wax paper, then on a baking sheet. Spray well with cooking spray. Bake for about 12 minutes at 400 degrees, flip half way through, and respray.

Low-fat packaged foods

When you see food with a "fat-free" or "low-fat" label, you may assume it's good for you. But chances are, they could put you at risk for heart disease. When manufacturers remove the fat from foods, like salad dressings, they add more sodium and sugar to the foods to make them taste good.

.Canned soup

If you enjoy soup, it's best to make your own instead of turning to the convenient cans you buy in the supermarket. If you don't want to make your own, be sure to read the label, as canned soup is often very high in sodium. Eating too much of this mineral can cause high blood pressure and heart disease.

8. Staying overweight

It's true that people who are overweight are at a greater risk of developing problems with their hearts. An even better way to judge if your weight may affect your heart is to measure your waist. People who carry fat in that area tend to develop heart-related complications more than those who carry it elsewhere on their bodies. It's recommended that men maintain a waist size of 40 inches or less. Women should aim for 35 inches or smaller.

9. Ignoring your body's warning signs

Finally, heart disease doesn't usually develop overnight. Your body often gives you warning signs. If you have high blood pressure, high blood sugar, high cholesterol, or a high resting heart rate, take steps to correct them.

Weight Loss

Weight loss is one of the most effective lifestyle changes you can make to control your blood pressure. Blood pressure often increases as weight increases. Being overweight can cause disrupted breathing during sleep (also known as sleep apnea), which raises blood pressure even further. Additionally, carrying too much weight around your waist (more than 40 inches for men and 35 inches for women) can put you at greater risk. Losing just 10 pounds can help reduce your blood pressure.

Regular Exercise

At least 30 minutes of regular physical activity most days of the week is one of the best ways to reduce high blood pressure. However, consistency is important here. If you stop exercising, your blood pressure can rise again. Some of the best types of exercise for reducing blood pressure are walking, jogging, cycling, swimming, dancing, or strength training. Consider joining a gym or taking a 30-minute walk each day.

Healthy Diet/Low Sodium

Eating whole grains, fruits, vegetables, and low-fat dairy products, as well as watching sodium intake, are easy ways to lower blood pressure. At the same time, try to cut down on saturated fats and cholesterol. For many of us, changing eating habits is easier said than done. A great way to spur positive change is to make a food diary. Start by writing down what you eat for one week to get a better picture of what you eat, how much, when, and why.

Additionally, aim to boost your potassium intake. Potassium can lessen the effects of sodium on blood pressure. In general, try to limit sodium to less than 2,300 mg a day. Even a small reduction in the sodium in your diet can lower your blood pressure. Be sure to read food labels when you shop and choose low-sodium alternatives and fewer processed foods. From there, avoid adding additional salt.

Limit alcohol consumption.

In small amounts, alcohol can potentially lower your blood pressure. But that protective effect is lost if you drink too much alcohol—more than one drink a day for women and men older than 65, or more than two drinks a day for men 65 and younger. One drink is the equivalent of 12 ounces of beer, five ounces of wine, or 1.5 ounces of 80-proof liquor. Drinking any more than these moderate amounts of alcohol can raise blood pressure by several points. Meanwhile, it also reduces the effectiveness of blood pressure medications.

Find ways to reduce stress.

Chronic stress is a big contributor to high blood pressure. Even occasional stress can contribute to high blood pressure if you react to stress by eating unhealthy food, drinking alcohol, or smoking. Examine the causes of your stress. Is it family, work, finances, or illness? Once you determine what's causing your stress, you can take steps to eliminate or reduce it.

Once you start making lifestyle changes, we recommend monitoring your blood pressure at home. And while making major changes can be beneficial, it's often just as effective to make changes one small step at a time. Try just one of these easy ways to lower blood pressure, and then, after you do it consistently, add in another one.

Chapter 4

Heart's health and longevity

How to keep your heart healthy as you get older is a really important question. You've got to try to avoid coronary heart disease to start with.

There is an epidemic of heart failure in our community in America, and that's because we've allowed our hearts to age more than they should. And there are all sorts of reasons why your heart ages. One is that your blood pressure's been too high. The second is your diet. You've not had as diverse a diet as you should, with lots of red vegetables, olive oil, and so on. Cuisine that's like the Mediterranean cuisine, which provides what are called bioactive compounds in your diet. These compounds stop the biological rusting and ageing of your cardiovascular system.

The best way, though, to prevent ageing of your heart and weakness of the muscles in the long term is exercise. This is best done as early in life as you can possibly do it. And even at older ages, starting to exercise is a really good idea. You've just got to do it steadily. But intense exercise, as intense as you're able or allowed to do, with muscle strengthening, will strengthen the heart muscle and make it beat more efficiently.

In June 2022, the American Heart Association updated the metrics for optimal cardiovascular health to include sleep—Life's_Essential. The tool measures four indicators related to cardiovascular and metabolic health status (blood pressure, cholesterol, blood sugar, and body mass index) and four behavioral and lifestyle factors (smoking status, physical activity, sleep, and diet).

"These two abstracts really give us some nice new insight into how we can understand at different stages across the life course just how important focusing on your cardiovascular health is going to be, particularly using the new American Heart Association's Essential 8 metrics," said Donald M. Lloyd-Jones, M.D.,

Sc.M., FAHA. Lloyd-Jones led the advisory writing group for Life's Essential 8 and is immediate past president of the American Heart Association, chair of the department of preventive medicine, the Eileen M. Foell Professor of Heart Research, and professor of preventive medicine, medicine, and pediatrics at Northwestern University's Feinberg School of Medicine in Chicago. "The cardiovascular health construct studied in these two abstracts really does nail what patients are trying to do, which is find the fountain of youth. Yes, live longer, but more importantly, live healthier longer, and extend that health span so that you can really enjoy quality in your remaining life years."

Life's Essential 8 and Life Expectancy Free of Cardiovascular Disease, Diabetes, Cancer, and Dementia in Adults

The first study investigated whether levels of cardiovascular health estimated by the

Association's Life's Essential metrics were associated with life expectancy free of major chronic diseases, including cardiovascular disease, type 2 diabetes, cancer, and dementia.

"Our study looked at the association between life's essentials and life expectancy free of major chronic disease in adults in the United Kingdom," said lead author Xuan Wang, M.D., Ph.D., a postdoctoral fellow and biostatistician in the department of epidemiology at Tulane University's School of Public Health and Tropical Medicine in New Orleans.

"We categorized Life's Essential scores according to the American Heart Association's recommendations, with scores of less than 50 out of 100 being poor cardiovascular health, 50 to less than 80 being intermediate, and 80 and above being ideal," Wang said. Life's Essential 8 scores of

80 and above are defined as "high cardiovascular health" by the Association.

When the researchers compared life expectancy and disease-free years among the groups, they found:

- Adults who scored as having ideal cardiovascular health lived substantially longer than those in the poor heart health category. Men and women with ideal cardiovascular health at age 50 had an average 5.2 years and 6.3 years more of total life expectancy, respectively, when compared to the men and women who scored as having poor cardiovascular health.

- Adults with ideal cardiovascular health scores lived longer without chronic disease. Disease-free life expectancy accounted for nearly 76% of total life expectancy for men.

- And more than 83% for women who had ideal cardiovascular health; in contrast, disease-free life expectancy was only 64.9% for men and 69.4% for women with poor cardiovascular health.

"Moreover, we found disparities in disease-free life expectancy due to low socioeconomic status may be offset considerably by maintaining an ideal cardiovascular health score in all adults," Wang said. "Our findings may stimulate interest in individual self-assessment and motivate people to improve their cardiovascular health. These findings support improving population health by promoting adherence to ideal cardiovascular health, which may also narrow health disparities related to socioeconomic status."

The study's limitations were that the researchers only included CVD, diabetes, cancer, and dementia in their definition of "disease-free life expectancy;" information on e-cigarettes was not available in the U.K. Biobank, which may lead to a slight overestimation of the LE8 score in this study; and participants in the U.K. Biobank are overwhelmingly white race; therefore, further studies are needed to confirm if these results are consistent among people from diverse racial and ethnic backgrounds who may experience negative social determinants of health throughout their lifetime.

"What's really important is that people maintaining high cardiovascular health into midlife are avoiding those chronic diseases of ageing—things like cancer and dementia—that we also worry about, not just cardiovascular disease," Lloyd-Jones said. "They're delayed until much later in the lifespan, so people can enjoy the life in their years as well as the years in their life."

A healthy heart is central to overall good health. Embracing a healthy lifestyle at any age can prevent heart disease and lower your risk of a heart attack or stroke. You are never too old or too young to begin taking care of your heart. True, the younger you begin making healthy choices, the longer you can reap the benefits. But swapping good habits for bad to promote good health can make a difference, even if you've already suffered a heart attack.

Choosing healthier foods and exercising are two of the best ways to contribute to good heart health. There are additional things you can do to lower your risk of heart disease.

Cardiovascular diseases have high rates of morbidity, mortality, and disability and are the leading causes of human death, irrespective of age, race, and region. According to the World Heart Federation, one-third of adults over the age of 25 suffer from cardiovascular diseases globally. Every year, over 17.5 million people die from cardiovascular diseases worldwide, which contributes to 30 percent of the annual death rate. The prognosis of cardiovascular diseases has been greatly improved in recent years with the development of medical technologies, leading to a decrease in morbidity and mortality. However, the morbidity and mortality due to heart diseases in developing countries are increasing, mainly due to environmental factors and unhealthy living habits. A great deal of attention is required to lead a healthy lifestyle and create an unpolluted environment to benefit the lives and health of our hearts.

Smoking cessation: Smoking is closely associated with various cardiovascular diseases, including coronary heart disease and hypertension. Compared with non-smokers, the risk of cardiovascular diseases for smokers increases 1.6 fold. A report from the

Asia Pacific Cohort Studies Collaboration indicates that smokers are 27 percent more likely to develop ischemic heart disease, 9 percent more likely to have hemorrhagic stroke, 4.5 times more likely to have hypertension, and 16 times more likely to have hyperlipidemia. Studies suggest that the risk of myocardial infarction for non-smokers who live with smokers increases by 23 percent. Summary analysis shows that in a person who has no history of cardiovascular disease, smoking cessation reduced the mortality of cardiovascular disease by about 2–35%, which is similar to the effect of antihypertensive intervention. Cessation before the age of 40 reduces the risk of death associated with continued smoking by about 90 percent. [6]. For those who have heart disease, quitting smoking can reduce overall mortality by 12–35 percent. This effect is significantly better than antihypertensive and lipid-lowering treatments.

Diet: Diet is crucial in the development and prevention of cardiovascular disease and is one of the key factors that one can change for a healthy heart. Abnormal blood lipid levels have been shown to have a strong correlation with the risk of coronary heart disease, and the abnormal blood lipid levels are directly related to the diet. A diet rich in saturated fats often causes high serum cholesterol levels. Unsaturated fats, like those found in fish, nuts, seeds, and vegetables, are beneficial for the heart. These sources of unsaturated fats contain essential fatty acids, including omega-3 and omega-6, which are beneficial to the heart and cannot be produced by the body.

Hypertension is another important risk factor for cardiovascular diseases, which is partly attributed to a high-sodium diet. The daily intake of salt should be less than 5 g, according to the recommendations of the WHO.

Unhealthy diets, including fast food, increase the risk of hypercholesterolemia, hypertension, and diabetes, which ultimately damage the heart. To keep a healthy heart, it is necessary to have a diet low in saturated fats and salt but with plenty of fresh fruit and vegetables.

Exercise: Exercise can influence a variety of cardiovascular regulatory peptides, lower C-reactive protein (CRP) levels, and delay the development of cardiovascular diseases. Exercise can reduce body fat levels and improve insulin sensitivity. Sticking to a long-term exercise regimen is an effective method to reduce CRP, and both help prevent cardiovascular disease. Milani and colleagues compared the effects of cardiovascular rehabilitation training for three months in 235 coronary heart disease patients with 42 patients with no rehabilitation therapy. The results showed that the body fat index, motility, and other cardiovascular risk factors were significantly improved in the rehabilitated group.

Pollution Control: It is suggested that environmental pollution is a greater cause of congenital heart disease than genetic factors. The development of the foetus is also influenced by a polluted environment during pregnancy, which can ultimately lead to congenital heart disease. Although the epidemiological evidence is limited and inconsistencies remain, recent studies have suggested that maternal exposure to air pollution may also play a role in causing congenital anomalies, particularly congenital heart diseases.

The impact of pollution from the environment has been studied on 45 heart disease patients in an area of Helsinki, Finland. Volunteers in the trial dramatically reduced the amount of blood flow into the heart after breathing polluted air for just two days. Though there was no pain associated with this change in heart function, it was a hallmark of heart disease progression. Epidemiological studies corroborate the elevated risk for cardiovascular events associated with exposure to PM2.5. $PM_{2.5}$ has been associated with increased risks of myocardial infarction, stroke, arrhythmia, and heart failure exacerbation within hours to days of exposure in susceptible individuals.

In conclusion, cardiovascular diseases are a devastating set of diseases that are best combated by preventative measures, including a healthy diet and a healthy lifestyle. Government agencies and individuals around the world should work together to create societies that promote the pursuit of a healthy heart and a happy life.

Mental wellness has been shown to be closely connected to the health of your heart. Stress, depression, anxiety, anger, and social isolation can all affect your cardiovascular health.

There are simple ways that you can promote mental wellness and reduce stress in your life, which will help you manage your heart health as well:

- Regular exercise

- Practicing mindfulness

- Connecting with others to reduce social isolation

- Getting professional help for mental wellness

How can exercise improve my mental and physical wellness?

Regular physical activity has been shown to reduce stress and positively affect your mental wellness. You might be surprised to find that when you start moving, you may have more self-confidence, experience better sleep, see a reduction in symptoms of depression and anxiety, and have the energy to engage in more social interaction and activities.

Finding an activity that you can integrate into your current lifestyle is key to starting and maintaining regular physical activity. Examples of physical activity can include going for regular walks, biking, and swimming, dancing, practicing yoga, joining a team sport, playing golf, lifting weights, or engaging in a seasonal activity such as snowshoeing or paddle boarding.

Learn more about integrating exercise and activity into your daily life from the Heart and Stroke Foundation and the American Heart Association.

How does practicing mindfulness work to improve my mental wellness?

Practicing mindfulness is another way to promote mental wellness by reducing stress, promoting sleep, and helping you feel more balanced and connected. There is growing evidence that practicing mindfulness may contribute to reducing the risk of heart disease and stroke.

Mindfulness is defined as the basic human ability to be fully present, aware of where we are and what we're doing, and not overly reactive or overwhelmed by what's going on around us. Mindfulness can be practiced through meditation, utilizing physical relaxation techniques, and breathing exercises.

To learn how you may integrate mindfulness into your daily life, read here to Help's mindfulness module and the BC Crisis Centre's mindfulness tools.

How does reducing social isolation work to improve my risk of heart disease?

Social isolation and loneliness have been linked to an increased risk of coronary heart disease. Meaningful social interactions and support may act as a preventative measure for the heart by reducing chronic stress and unhealthy coping strategies, which are often associated with loneliness.

If you are looking to reduce social isolation and increase your social support, you can try:

- Developing a new hobby

- Volunteering in the community

- Joining a community or neighborhood group

- Joining a book club, gardening club, or hiking club

- Enrolling in a course to learn a new skill

- Joining an exercise class or sports team

- Connecting online with family and old or new friends

Learn about more ways to expand your social connections and reduce isolation.

When should I seek professional help to maintain my mental wellness?

If you continue to find it challenging to manage your stress or are experiencing symptoms of depression and/or anxiety, it may be time to seek professional support and help. You can start by speaking with your family doctor or connecting with a local counsellor to discuss coping strategies to manage your stress. Counselling services may be covered or partially covered by your extended health benefits.

The first and most obvious reason is that heart disease is deadly. More people die from heart disease in the U.S. than all cancers combined, and that includes men and women. It's the number one killer of adults in the U.S., and it has been for decades. Tragically, the American Heart Association says that 82 percent of Americans know heart attacks can be prevented but don't do anything about it. And 72 percent of Americans don't think they're at risk for heart disease. Considering the fact that obesity is a risk factor and 42.4 percent of Americans struggle with obesity, it's very unlikely that 72 percent of Americans exhibit no risk factors. In fact, nearly half of American adults have already been diagnosed with some form of cardiovascular disease, according to a 2019 issue of the journal Circulation.

The American Heart Association also reports that 2,300 people die from cardiovascular disease (stroke and heart disease) every day. Even more tragic, 80 percent of these deaths are preventable through lifestyle changes. We have to take these statistics seriously if we want to lower them and live longer, healthier lives.

Heart disease affects your mental health.

A second reason to care about your heart health is because it affects your mental health. A recent survey conducted by the British Heart Foundation's Heart Matters Magazine found that 68 percent of people with heart disease said their condition had affected them mentally, emotionally, or psychologically.

This impact on mental health largely stems from fear and anxiety around having a heart attack, stroke, or cardiac arrest, which also encompasses the effect those events would have on loved ones. Many people with heart conditions are worried about leaving their children or spouses without support. Even more concerning is the fact that in this survey, 67 percent of those people whose mental health had been negatively impacted by heart disease said they didn't talk to anyone about it.

Not only is it important to keep yourself healthy to prevent a medical emergency, but it also minimizes the likelihood of experiencing the emotional and mental toll that can come along with a diagnosis.

Heart disease is largely preventable but not reversible.

Remember that 80 percent of strokes and heart disease are preventable, even though heart disease is the number one killer of adults in the U.S. Though you can live with heart disease and often prevent further damage, there is no cure. Once plaque begins to build up in your arteries, for example, it will not go away on its own with diet and lifestyle changes. In severe cases, a doctor may recommend removing the plaque surgically, but in most cases, the priority is to prevent further buildup.

In addition to eating a balanced diet and getting regular exercise, keeping tabs on your body is crucial to prevention. Getting regular checkups and staying in touch with your general practitioner is important, and if you exhibit any risk factors, getting screened for cardiovascular diseases could save your life. Screenings are simple and non-invasive, and they can tell you whether or not you have plaque buildup in your arteries or show signs of atrial fibrillation (an irregular heartbeat) and other cardiac issues.

It's a good idea to talk to your doctor about getting screened if you exhibit any of these risk factors:

- Age 50+

- Family history of heart disease or stroke

- Obesity

- High blood pressure

- High cholesterol

- Diabetes

- Smoking

Stay informed and prevent heart disease.

As always, staying informed about your health is the number one key to prevention. Life Line Screening provides quick, painless screenings for atrial fibrillation, carotid artery disease, peripheral artery disease, and more. Schedule a screening today to arm yourself with knowledge about your own health so you can be better equipped to live the life you want to live.

Chapter 5

How are conditions of the heart diagnosed?

Your health care provider will examine you and ask about your personal and family medical history.

Many different tests are used to diagnose heart disease. Besides blood tests and a chest X-ray, tests to diagnose heart disease can include:

- **Electrocardiogram (ECG or EKG)** An ECG is a quick and painless test that records the electrical signals in the heart. It can tell if the heart is beating too fast or too slowly.

- **Holter monitoring.** A Holter monitor is a portable ECG device that's worn for a day or more to record the heart's activity during daily activities. This test can detect irregular heartbeats that aren't found during a regular ECG exam.

- This noninvasive exam uses sound waves to create detailed images of the heart in motion. It shows how blood moves through the heart and heart valves. An echocardiogram can help determine if a valve is narrowed or leaking.

- **Exercise tests or stress tests** these tests often involve walking on a treadmill or riding a stationary bike while the heart is monitored. Exercise tests help reveal how the heart responds to physical activity and whether heart disease symptoms occur during exercise. If you can't exercise, you might be given medications.

- **Cardiac catheterization.** This test can show blockages in the heart arteries. A long, thin, flexible tube (catheter) is inserted in a blood vessel, usually in the groyne or wrist, and guided to the heart. Dye flows through the catheter to the arteries in the heart. The dye helps the arteries show up more clearly on X-ray images taken during the test.

- **Heart (cardiac) CT scan** in a cardiac CT scan, you lie on a table inside a doughnut-shaped machine. An X-ray tube inside the machine rotates around your body and collects images of your heart and chest.

- **Heart (cardiac) magnetic resonance imaging (MRI) scan.** A cardiac MRI uses a magnetic field and computer-generated radio waves to create detailed images of the heart.

. Treatment

Heart disease treatment depends on the cause and type of heart damage. Healthy lifestyle habits—such as eating a low-fat, low-salt diet, getting regular exercise and good sleep, and not smoking—are an important part of treatment.

. Medications

If lifestyle changes alone don't work, medications may be needed to control heart disease symptoms and prevent complications. The type of medication used depends on the type of heart disease.

. Surgery or other procedures

Some people with heart disease may need a procedure or surgery. The type of procedure or surgery will depend on the type of heart disease and the amount of damage to the heart.

Diagnoses for coronary artery **and vascular disease**

An angiogram is a test that takes X-ray pictures of the coronary arteries and the vessels that supply blood to the heart. During an angiogram, a special dye is released into the coronary arteries from a catheter (special tube) inserted in a blood vessel. This dye makes the blood vessels visible when an X-ray is taken. Angiography allows doctors to clearly see how blood flows into the heart. This allows them to pinpoint problems with the coronary arteries.

Angiography may be recommended for patients with angina (chest pain) or those with suspected coronary artery disease (CAD). The test gives doctors valuable information on the condition of the coronary arteries, such as atherosclerosis, regurgitation (blood flowing backwards through the heart valves), or pooling of blood in a chamber because of a valve malfunction.

What should I expect?

Angiography is performed in a hospital or clinic. You will be asked to lie on a table, and the site where the catheter is to be inserted (the groyne or arm) will be cleaned. You will be given a local an aesthetic to numb the skin so you feel no pain. Then, a catheter is carefully guided through a vein or artery to a position near the heart. When the catheter is in place, it releases a special dye into the bloodstream. While the dye is being released, you might feel a brief sensation of heat, which usually passes quickly. An angiogram can take about one to two hours. However, it is best to check with the center where you are having the procedure to find out how long it will take.

Angiography is a very common procedure and is generally considered safe. In some patients, the contrast dye may cause nausea, the need to urinate, or even allergic reactions, although these side effects are rare.

How to prepare

Generally, you should not eat or drink for 6 to 8 hours before having a coronary angiography.

Echocardiogram

An echocardiogram (ECHO) uses sound waves (ultrasound) to create a picture of your heart. The recorded waves show the shape, texture, and movement of your heart valves, as well as the size of your heart chambers and how well they are working. An ECHO may be done to assess a variety of heart conditions, such as heart murmurs, damage to heart muscle in those who have had a heart attack, and infections in the heart. It may also be recommended if you are experiencing abnormal heart sounds, shortness of breath, palpitations, angina (chest pain), or have a history of stroke. It is very useful in diagnosing heart valve problems.

What to expect

A gel is placed on your chest to help transmit the sound waves, and a transducer (a unit that directs sound waves) is moved over your chest. This test involves no pain or discomfort. A typical test takes about 15 to 45 minutes.

How to prepare

For a regular echocardiogram, no special preparation is needed. If you have questions, it is best to check with the center where you are having your test for specific information about how to prepare.

Electrocardiogram (ECG/EKG)

What is an ECG or an EKG? An electrocardiogram (ECG or EKG) is a test that checks how your heart is functioning by measuring the electrical activity of the heart. With each heartbeat, an electrical impulse (or wave) travels through your heart. This wave causes the muscle to squeeze and pump blood from the heart.

An ECG measures and records the electrical activity that passes through the heart. A doctor can determine if this electrical activity is normal or irregular.

An ECG may be recommended if you are experiencing arrhythmia, chest pain, or palpitations, and an abnormal ECG result can be a signal of a number of different heart conditions.

Why is it done?

- To detect abnormal heart rhythms that may have caused blood clots to form.

- Detect heart problems, including a recent or ongoing heart attack, abnormal heart rhythms (arrhythmias), coronary artery blockage, areas of damaged heart muscle (from a prior heart attack), enlargement of the heart, and inflammation of the sac surrounding the heart (pericarditis).

- Detect non-heart conditions such as electrolyte imbalances and lung diseases.

- Monitor recovery from a heart attack, the progression of heart disease, or the effectiveness of certain heart medications or a pacemaker.

- Rule out hidden heart disease in patients about to undergo surgery.

How do you prepare?

You do not have to restrict what you eat or drink before your ECG, although it is recommended that you not smoke just before the test. You will be asked to remove your jewellery and wear a hospital gown.

What can you expect?

- An ECG is a non-invasive procedure, which means that nothing is injected into the body.

- It is painless.

- A number of electrodes—usually a total of 12 to 15—are attached to various locations on your body, including your arm, leg, and chest.

- The electrodes are attached by small suction cups or adhesive patches.

- Sensors in the pads detect the electrical activity of your heart.

- The test is usually performed while you lie still.

- Results are most often recorded on graph paper and interpreted or read by your doctor or a technologist.

- The test usually takes 5 to 10 minutes.

Exercise electrocardiogram

What is a stress test?

An exercise electrocardiogram (ECG) records your heart's response to the stress of exercise. An exercise ECG measures your heart's electrical activity, blood pressure, and heart rate while you exercise, usually by walking on a treadmill.

Why is it done?

- A stress test is usually done to pinpoint the cause of unexplained chest pain, especially if coronary artery disease (heart disease) is suspected.

- If you have been diagnosed with coronary artery disease, you may be given an exercise ECG to determine how far the disease has progressed and how much exercise you can do safely.

- If you have had a heart attack or heart surgery, it can help determine how much work or exercise you can do safely.

- It may also be recommended if you are experiencing irregular heartbeats (arrhythmia), very fast or slow heartbeats (tachycardia or bradycardia), palpitations (unusual throbbing or fluttering sensations in the heart), dizziness, or excessive fatigue.

How do you prepare?

- Wear clothing and shoes that are comfortable for exercising.

- You'll probably be told not to eat for at least two hours before the test.

- If you're a smoker, you'll also need to not smoke for at least two hours before the test.

What can you expect?

- An exercise ECG is usually done in a clinic or hospital.

- You will be asked to walk on a treadmill (or sometimes pedal a stationary bicycle).

- If small metal electrodes are attached to your chest, then you will either begin by walking slowly or pedaling.

- As you walk, a technician will monitor your heart's activity and rate, your breathing, and your blood pressure.

- Gradually, the speed of the treadmill increases, so you have to walk more quickly. This will help your doctor see how your heart handles progressively greater challenges.

- The test continues until your heart is beating as fast as it safely can (you reach your peak exercise capacity, given your age and condition) or until you experience chest pain.

- It is generally a safe procedure, although it may trigger chest pain or irregular heart rhythms. Be sure to let someone know if you are feeling any discomfort or other symptoms.

- The length of time for the test is usually between 15 and 30 minutes.

Thallium or cardio lite scan

What is a thallium scan or a cardio lite scan?

A thallium (or cardio lite) scan uses a radioactive tracer to see how much blood is reaching different parts of your heart. These tests are the more common forms of tests called nuclear medicine scans. You may also hear them called:

- thallium myocardial imaging

- Cold spot imaging

- Myocardial perfusion imaging

- Thallium scintigraphy.

Why it's done

- These scans are often done to determine the size and location of injured muscle after a heart attack and will help your doctor find out more about your heart's cells and its blood supply.

- It is also sometimes done after bypass surgery to see whether grafted blood vessels are functioning properly.

- It may be recommended for people with persistent, unexplained chest pain or to learn more about irregularities found during an **electrocardiogram (ECG or EKG)**.

How do you prepare?

You will probably be told not to eat or drink for at least three hours before your test or to abstain from having any tobacco, alcohol, caffeinated beverages, or over-the-counter medications in the 24 hours before the procedure.

Be sure to talk to your doctor if you have diabetes, discuss any prescription medications you are taking, and if you have any allergies.

It is best to check with the center where you are having your test for specific information about how to prepare.

What can you expect?

- You will be asked to lie on a table, and then a small amount of thallium (a radioactive tracer) is injected into a vein in your arm.

- A special camera then measures the amount of tracer that is carried through your bloodstream into your heart.

- The parts of your heart that receive a good blood supply will pick up the tracer.

- The areas with poor blood supply will not pick it up, so they will appear as dark areas (cold spots) on the scan.

- Thallium scans may sometimes be done after exercise. It is best to check with the center where you are having the test to find out how long the scan will take.

This is a relatively low-risk procedure. The amount of radiation absorbed by your body during this test is about the same as from a CT scan.

Travel advice

Talk to your doctor before scheduling any travel plans shortly after your scan. With increased security at airports and border crossings, sophisticated scanning techniques may detect small amounts of residual radiation in your body, which could lead to travel delays. Your doctor will help you determine how and when to schedule your travel following your scan.

Diagnoses for heart rhythm disorders

(Arrhythmia)

Electrophysiology Study

What is EPS?

An electrophysiology study (EPS) is a test that helps determine what kind of arrhythmia (irregular heartbeat) you have and what can be done to control it. Not everyone with an abnormal heartbeat needs an EPS, and many people may just be given an electrocardiogram (ECG/EKG).

What to expect

Special catheters (thin flexible tubes) are inserted through a vein in your arm, groyne, or neck and guided to your heart to record its electrical activity. You will be asked to lie on a special table and be monitored by an ECG machine. An intravenous (IV) will be attached, and the site where the catheters are to be inserted will be cleaned. You will then be given a local an aesthetic to numb the skin so you feel no pain. Then, the catheters will be carefully guided through a vein into the right side of the heart.

You will be given controlled electrical impulses to see how your heart reacts. For example, if you are prone to rapid heartbeats (tachycardia), these may be deliberately triggered during the procedure so that your doctor can see how it affects your heart. Medications may also be tested to see which ones will stop the arrhythmia. Once the electrical pathways causing the arrhythmia are found, radio waves can be sent through the catheter to destroy them (ablation). A diagnostic electrophysiology study takes approximately 1 to 2 hours, and an ablation may take an additional 1 to 4 hours. You will be returned to your room, where you will be monitored and required to rest for approximately 4 to 6 hours.

When your heart receives the electrical impulses to make it beat at different speeds, you may feel slightly uncomfortable. After the doctors have the information they need, the catheter and IV will be removed. After an EPS, you'll be asked to lie down for a few hours. You may eat or drink immediately after.

How to prepare

You will probably be told not to eat or drink anything after midnight the night before your test. If you have diabetes or are taking any medications, talk to your doctor to find out if you need to make any special preparations.

Holter or event monitoring

What is Holter monitoring?

Holter monitoring is usually used to diagnose heart rhythm disturbances, specifically to find the cause of palpitations or dizziness.

You wear a small recording device called a Holter monitor, which is connected to small metal discs (called electrodes) that are placed on your chest to get a reading of your heart rate and rhythm over a 24-hour period or longer. Your heart's rhythm is transmitted and recorded on a tape, then played back into a computer so it can be analyzed to find out what is causing your arrhythmia. Some monitors let you push a record button to capture a rhythm as soon as you feel any symptoms.

What is event monitoring?

Like a Holter monitor, an event recorder also uses a recording device to monitor your heart, although it uses a smaller monitoring device. Unlike the Holter, it does not continuously monitor your heart over a 24-hour period. It doesn't record until you feel symptoms and trigger the monitor.

When you feel the symptoms of an arrhythmia, you can telephone a monitoring station, where a record can be made. Or, if you cannot get to a phone, you can save the information on the event monitor, which can later be sent to a monitoring station.

A cardiac event recorder is also called a loop monitor or a patient-activated ECG.

What to expect

Setting up the monitor only takes a few minutes, and then you can go about your regular daily activities.

You may be asked to write down any symptoms you have while wearing the monitor so your heartbeat at that particular time can later be analyzed.

How to prepare

It is best to check with the center where you are having your test for specific information about how to prepare.

Tilt table exam

Why is a tilt-table exam done?

Tilt tests are especially useful if you have been fainting without any explanation. These tests help doctors understand how your body posture affects your blood pressure. The goal is to find out if different drugs or different body positions will trigger an arrhythmia (an abnormal heartbeat) or other symptoms.

What to expect

In this test, you are asked to lie on a special bed that can be tilted to different positions. You will be safely strapped in. Your heart and blood pressure will be monitored throughout the test. An IV (an intravenous line or tube) is put into a vein in your arm so you can receive different drugs during the test. Then, the bed you are lying on is tilted so that you go from a reclining position to an almost upright one. At the same time, you may be given drugs through the IV. Some of these medications may cause side effects such as stomach aches, nausea, lightheadedness, or a rapid heartbeat. These effects do not last long. Your reactions will often help your doctor pinpoint the exact cause of your arrhythmia. The test varies by patient and usually lasts anywhere from 30 minutes to two hours.

How to prepare

Your doctor will talk to you about what you can eat and drink before the test. He or she will also tell you if and how to adjust any medications you may be taking. It is best to check with the center where you are having your test for specific information about how to prepare.

Valvular heart disease diagnosis

Tests for valvular heart disease also include:

Angiography or arteriography

What is it?

An angiogram is a test that takes X-ray pictures of the coronary arteries and the vessels that supply blood to the heart. During an angiogram, a special dye is released into the coronary arteries from a catheter (special tube) inserted in a blood vessel. This dye makes the blood vessels visible when an X-ray is taken. Angiography allows doctors to clearly see how blood flows into the heart.

This allows them to pinpoint problems with the coronary arteries.

Angiography may be recommended for patients with angina (chest pain) or those with suspected coronary artery disease (CAD). The test gives doctors valuable information on the condition of the coronary arteries, such as atherosclerosis, regurgitation (blood flowing backwards through the heart valves), or pooling of blood in a chamber because of a valve malfunction.

What should I expect?

Angiography is performed in a hospital or clinic. You will be asked to lie on a table, and the site where the catheter is to be inserted (the groyne or arm) will be cleaned. You will be given a local an aesthetic to numb the skin so you feel no pain. Then, a catheter is carefully guided through a vein or artery to a position near the heart. When the catheter is in place, it releases a special dye into the bloodstream. While the dye is being released, you might feel a brief sensation of heat, which usually passes quickly. An angiogram can take about one to two hours. However, it is best to check with the center where you are having the procedure to find out how long it will take.

Angiography is a very common procedure and is generally considered safe. In some patients, the contrast dye may cause nausea, the need to urinate, or even allergic reactions, although these side effects are rare.

How to prepare

Generally, you should not eat or drink for 6 to 8 hours before having a coronary angiography. Speak to your doctor about how to prepare for the test, specifically about food, drink, and medications. If you have questions, it is best to check with the center where you are having your test for specific information about how to prepare.

Chest X-ray

What is a chest X-ray?

A chest X-ray is a picture of the heart, lungs, and bones of the chest.

Why is it done?

A chest X-ray can help your doctor determine if your heart is an unusual shape or if it is larger than it should be. It can also help confirm the presence of a valve disorder and provide important, detailed information about your condition and its seriousness. Chest X-rays are useful for diagnosing an enlargement of the heart (cardiomyopathy) or heart failure.

What can you expect?

- No special preparation is necessary.

- Having chest X-rays is completely painless and only takes a few minutes.

- Wearing a hospital gown, you will be asked to lie on an X-ray table, and a technologist will help to position you properly.

- You will have to hold your breath and lie very still for two to three seconds.

- The X-ray machine is turned on briefly, letting a small beam of X-rays pass through your chest to create an image on special X-ray film.

- Sometimes two pictures are taken—a front and side view.

- The X-ray film takes about 10 minutes to develop.

Heart MRI (Magnetic Resonance Imaging)

What is an MRI?

Magnetic resonance imaging (MRI) is a large imaging device that sits in its own room. It uses a harmless magnetic field and radio waves to get clear, sharp pictures of your heart and major blood vessels.

MRI images show even more detail than CT scans and can be viewed in 3-D on a computer screen.

Why it's done

Heart MRI is used to diagnose many diseases and conditions, including:

- Coronary artery disease

- Damage from a heart attack

- Heart failure

- Valve disorders

- Congenital heart disease

- Pericarditis

- Cardiac tumor's

What you can expect

- You will lie on a flat bed and then be moved inside the opening of the MRI device.

- The procedure will take approximately 30 minutes.

- You may find it difficult to stay motionless for that length of time, but the procedure itself is painless.

Heart failure diagnosis

Blood test and urine test

1. **Blood test**

Depending on what your doctor is looking for, any of the following may be tested:

- How smoothly your blood flows through your vessels.

- The time it takes for your blood to clot, as well as the level of a clotting component called fibrinogen,

- Your blood cholesterol levels

- Your blood sugar (glucose) level

- Your blood calcium levels

- Your blood hemoglobin levels

- Liver function

- Thyroid function

- Renal function

It is important to know that although blood tests can indicate your risk of having heart disease or other health conditions, often other confirmatory tests are needed to diagnose many diseases.

What is involved?

No special preparation is needed. Blood is drawn from a vein in one arm.

- Your arm is first cleaned with an antiseptic.

- A tourniquet (an elastic band) or a blood pressure cuff is placed around the upper arm, which causes the veins in the lower arm to fill with blood.

- A needle is inserted into the vein, and the blood is collected in a vial or syringe.

- Once blood is taken, the needle is removed, and a bandage is applied.

2. Urine test

Although it isn't always possible at the time of your initial examination, a simple urine test can help your doctor diagnose conditions related to stroke, including blood clots, kidney disease, other metabolic diseases, or diabetes.

What is involved?

You will be given a container to collect a sample. Try to collect your sample "midstream." As you start to urinate, allow a small amount to fall into the toilet bowl. Then, catch about 1 to 2 ounces (30 to 60 mL) and remove the container from the urine stream.

Angiography or arteriography

What is it?

An angiogram is a test that takes X-ray pictures of the coronary arteries and the vessels that supply blood to the heart. During an angiogram, a special dye is released into the coronary arteries from a catheter (special tube) inserted in a blood vessel. This dye makes the blood vessels visible when an X-ray is taken. Angiography allows doctors to clearly see how blood flows into the heart. This allows them to pinpoint problems with the coronary arteries.

Angiography may be recommended for patients with angina (chest pain) or those with suspected coronary artery disease (CAD). The test gives doctors valuable information on the condition of the coronary arteries, such as atherosclerosis, regurgitation (blood flowing backwards through the heart valves), or pooling of blood in a chamber because of a valve malfunction.

What should I expect?

Angiography is performed in a hospital or clinic. You will be asked to lie on a table, and the site where the catheter is to be inserted (the groyne or arm) will be cleaned. You will be given a local an aesthetic to numb the skin so you feel no pain. Then, a catheter is carefully guided through a vein or artery to a position near the heart. When the catheter is in place, it releases a special dye into the bloodstream. While the dye is being released, you might feel a brief sensation of heat, which usually passes quickly. An angiogram can take about one to two hours. However, it is best to check with the center where you are having the procedure to find out how long it will take.

Angiography is a very common procedure and is generally considered safe. In some patients, the contrast dye may cause nausea, the need to urinate, or even allergic reactions, although these side effects are rare.

How to prepare

Generally, you should not eat or drink for 6 to 8 hours before having a coronary angiography. Speak to your doctor about how to prepare for the test, specifically about food, drink, and medications. If you have questions, it is best to check with the center where you are having your test for specific information about how to prepare.

Chapter 6

Prevention and Risk Factors

As we see in the above chapter, it can be quite a challenge to deal with coronary artery disease, or CAD. It happens when plaque builds up in the walls of the arteries that supply the heart. These can narrow and cause chest pain (angina) and later a full-blown heart attack. But some people feel nothing at all until late into the disease.

CAD, also called heart disease or coronary heart disease, causes roughly 805,000 heart attacks and leads to 696,000 deaths each year in the U.S.

Because heart disease is so common and often goes silent until it strikes, it is important to recognize the factors that put you at risk.

What Raises Your Risk for Heart Disease?

There are risk factors for heart disease that you have control over and others that you don't. Uncontrollable risk factors for heart disease include:

- Being male

- Older age

- Family history of heart disease

- Being postmenopausal

- Race (African American, Native American, and Mexican American people are more likely to have heart disease)

Heart disease risk factors that you can control revolve around lifestyle. These include:

- Smoking

- Unhealthy cholesterol numbers (see below)

- Uncontrolled high blood pressure

- Physical inactivity

- Obesity (having a BMI greater than 25)

- Uncontrolled diabetes

- Uncontrolled stress, depression, and anger

- Poor diet

- Alcohol use

How Can You Lower Your Heart Disease Risk?

Research shows heart disease may be preventable more than half the time with simple lifestyle changes. Besides lowering your risk for heart attack and stroke, these changes can often improve your overall physical and mental health. Here are some ways you can change lifestyle factors to reduce your risk of heart disease:

Quit smoking. Smoking is the most preventable risk factor. Smokers have more than twice the risk of heart attack as nonsmokers and are much more likely to die from them. If you smoke, quit. Better yet, don't start smoking in the first place. Even if you don't smoke, constant exposure to other people's cigarette smoke (secondhand smoke) raises your risk of heart disease.

Improve cholesterol levels. Your risk for heart disease increases with unhealthy cholesterol numbers. The right levels can vary somewhat depending on your age, sex, overall health, and family health history. Ask your doctor about the right levels for you. In general, though, your levels should be as follows:

Total cholesterol: less than 200 mg/dL

"Good," or HDL, cholesterol: 60 mg/dL or greater

"Bad," or LDL, cholesterol: less than 100 mg/dL

Triglycerides: less than 150 mg/dL

A diet low in cholesterol, saturated and fats, and simple sugars and high in complex carbohydrates can help lower cholesterol levels in some people. Regular exercise will also help lower "bad" cholesterol and raise "good" cholesterol in some cases.

If that's not enough, your doctor may suggest a cholesterol medication, like a statin, to help lower levels.

Control high blood pressure. About 67 million people in the U.S. have high blood pressure, making it the most common risk factor for heart disease. Nearly 1 in 3 adults has systolic blood pressure (the upper number) over 130 and/or diastolic blood pressure (the lower number) over 80, which is the definition of high blood pressure. Your doctor will assess your blood pressure numbers in light of your overall health, lifestyle, and other risk factors. You and your doctor can come up with a plan to help control blood pressure through diet, exercise, weight management, and, if needed, medication.

Control diabetes. If not properly controlled, diabetes can lead to heart disease and heart damage, including heart attacks. Control diabetes through a healthy diet, exercise, maintaining a healthy weight, and medication as prescribed by your doctor.

Get active. People who don't exercise have higher rates of heart disease compared to people who perform even moderate amounts of physical activity. A bit of light gardening or walking can lower your risk of heart disease.

Most people should exercise 30 minutes a day, at moderate intensity, on most days. More vigorous exercise could help even more, but talk to your doctor first. Try to use large muscle groups and get your heart rate up. Aerobic activities that raise your heart rate include brisk walking, cycling, swimming, jumping rope, and jogging. You can also lift weights to increase strength and muscle endurance.

If motivation is a problem, make an exercise menu. Pick a couple of activities that sound like fun. That way, you always have some choices. Consult your doctor before starting any exercise program, especially if you have underlying health conditions or haven't exercised in a while.

Eat right. Eat a heart-healthy diet low in sodium, saturated fat, trans fat, cholesterol, and refined sugars. Try to increase your intake of foods rich in vitamins and other nutrients, especially antioxidants, which may lower your risk for heart disease. Also, eat plant-based foods such as fruits and vegetables, nuts, and whole grains.

Rethink your drink. Limit alcohol. Moderate drinking may be OK, but more than that isn't good for your heart health. What's moderate drinking? Up to one glass a day for women and up to two glasses a day for men

Maintain a healthy weight. Obesity by itself could raise your risk for heart disease. In addition, excess weight puts strain on your heart and often raises your risk of other heart disease risk factors like diabetes, high blood pressure, and high cholesterol. A balanced diet and regular exercise can help you maintain a healthy weight. Talk to your doctor if you need a safe plan for weight loss or if you want to figure out the right body weight for your heart health.

Manage stress. Poorly controlled stress and anger can worsen heart disease. Some approaches include:

Relaxation methods like meditation, tai chi, yoga, guided imagery, deep breathing, and other approaches

Talk therapy with a therapist or in a group setting for anger management, anxiety, or other issues

Time management. If you schedule your time carefully, you'll be less stressed about getting things done.

Realistic goal-setting. Think carefully about what you can realistically get done. If you promise too much to yourself or others, you may create stress when you're unable to deliver.

You know that a bad diet and too little exercise can hurt your ticker. But there are lots of sneaky sources of heart disease that you may not be aware of. Here are some things you need to know about and heart-smart steps to help you stay healthy.

Assessing the risk and protective factors that contribute to substance use disorders helps practitioner's select appropriate interventions. Many factors influence a person's chance of developing a mental and/or substance use disorder. Effective prevention focuses on reducing those risk factors and strengthening protective factors that are most closely related to the problem being addressed. Applying the Strategic Prevention Framework (SPF) helps prevention professionals identify factors having the greatest impact on their target population. Risk factors are characteristics at the biological, psychological, family, community, or cultural level that precede and are associated with a higher likelihood of negative outcomes. Protective factors are characteristics associated with a lower likelihood of negative outcomes or that reduce a risk factor's impact. Protective factors may be seen as positive countering events. Some risk and protective factors are fixed; they don't change over time. Other risk and protective factors are considered variable and can change over time. Variable risk factors include income level, peer group, adverse childhood experiences (ACEs), and employment status. Individual-level risk factors may include a person's genetic predisposition to addiction or exposure to alcohol prenatally. Individual-level protective factors might include positive self-image, self-control, or social competence.

Risk and protective factors are related, and

Cumulative

Risk factors tend to be positively correlated with one another and negatively correlated with protective factors. In other words, people with some risk factors have a greater chance of experiencing even more risk factors, and they are less likely to have protective factors.

Risk and protective factors also tend to have a cumulative effect on the development or reduced development of behavioral health issues. Young people with multiple risk factors have a greater likelihood of developing a condition that impacts their physical or mental health; young people with multiple protective factors are at a reduced risk.

These correlations underscore the importance of early intervention.

- Interventions that target multiple, not single, factors

All people have biological and psychological characteristics that make them vulnerable to, or resilient in the face of, potential behavioral health issues. Because people have relationships within their communities and larger society, each person's biological and psychological characteristics exist in multiple contexts. A variety of risk and protective factors operate within each of these contexts. These factors also influence each other.

Targeting only one context when addressing a person's risk or protective factors is unlikely to be successful because people don't exist in isolation. For example:

- In relationships, risk factors include parents who use drugs and alcohol or who suffer from mental illness, child abuse and maltreatment, and inadequate supervision. In this context, parental involvement is an example of a protective factor.

- In communities, risk factors include neighborhood poverty and violence. Here, protective factors could include the availability of faith-based resources and after

-school activities.

- In society, risk factors can include norms and laws favorable to substance use, as well as racism and a lack of economic opportunity. Protective factors in this context would include hate crime laws or policies limiting the availability of alcohol.

Prevention includes a wide range of activities—known as "interventions"—aimed at reducing risks or threats to health. You may have heard researchers and health experts talk about three categories of prevention: primary, secondary, and tertiary. What do they mean by these terms?

Primary prevention aims to prevent disease or injury before it ever occurs. This is done by preventing exposure to hazards that cause disease or injury, altering unhealthy or unsafe behaviors that can lead to disease or injury, and increasing resistance to disease or injury should exposure occur. Examples include:

- Legislation and enforcement to ban or control the use of hazardous products (e.g., asbestos) or to mandate safe and healthy practices (e.g., the use of seatbelts and bike helmets).

- education about healthy and safe habits (e.g., eating well, exercising regularly, not smoking)

- Immunization against infectious diseases.

Secondary prevention aims to reduce the impact of a disease or injury that has already occurred. This is done by detecting and treating disease or injury as soon as possible to halt or slow its progress, encouraging personal strategies to prevent reinjure or recurrence, and implementing programs to return people to their original health and function to prevent long-term problems. Examples include:

- Regular exams and screening tests to detect disease in its earliest stages (e.g., mammograms to detect breast cancer).

- daily, low-dose aspirins and/or diet and exercise programs to prevent further heart attacks or strokes

- Suitably modified work so injured or ill workers can return safely to their jobs.

Tertiary prevention aims to soften the impact of an ongoing illness or injury that has lasting effects. This is done by helping people manage long-term, often-complex health problems and injuries (e.g., chronic diseases, permanent impairments) in order to improve as much as possible their ability to function, their quality of life, and their life expectancy. Examples include:

- Cardiac or stroke rehabilitation programs, chronic disease management programs (e.g., for diabetes, arthritis, depression, etc.)

- Support groups that allow members to share strategies for living well.

- Vocational rehabilitation programs to retrain workers for new jobs when they have recovered as much as possible.

Part of learning how to take charge of your health requires understanding your risk factors for different diseases. Risk factors are things in your life that increase your chances of getting a certain disease. Some risk factors are beyond your control. You may be born with them or exposed to them through no fault of your own.

People with a family history of chronic disease may have the most to gain from making lifestyle changes. You can't change your genes, but you can change behaviors that affect your health, such as smoking, inactivity, and poor eating habits. In many cases, making these changes can reduce your risk of disease, even if the disease runs in your family. Another change you can make is to have screening tests, such as mammograms and colorectal cancer screening. These screening tests help detect disease early. People who have a family health history of a chronic disease may benefit the most from screening tests that look for risk factors or early signs of disease. Finding disease early, before symptoms appear, can mean better health in the long run.

Chapter 7

Treatments of heart disease

when we generalize, the treatments, as we see some of them above.

Heart disease treatment depends on the cause and type of heart damage. Healthy lifestyle habits—such as eating a low-fat, low-salt diet, getting regular exercise and good sleep, and not smoking—are an important part of treatment.

Medications

If lifestyle changes alone don't work, medications may be needed to control heart disease symptoms and prevent complications. The type of medication used depends on the type of heart disease.

Surgery or other procedures

Some people with heart disease may need a procedure or surgery. The type of procedure or surgery will depend on the type of heart disease and the amount of damage to the heart.

Lifestyle and home remedies

Heart disease can be improved—or even prevented—by making certain lifestyle changes. The following changes are recommended to improve heart health:

- **Don't smoke.** Smoking is a major risk factor for heart disease, especially atherosclerosis. Quitting is the best way to reduce the risk of heart disease and its complications. If you need help quitting, talk to your provider.

- **Eat healthy foods.** Eat plenty of fruits, vegetables, and whole grains. Limit sugar, salt, and saturated fats.

- **Control blood pressure.** Uncontrolled high blood pressure increases the risk of serious health problems. Get your blood pressure checked at least every two years if you're 18 and older. If you have risk factors for heart disease or are over age 40, you may need more frequent checks. Ask your health care provider what blood pressure reading is best for you.

- **Get a cholesterol test.** Ask your provider for a baseline cholesterol test when you're in your 20s and then at least every 4 to 6 years. You may need to start testing earlier if high cholesterol is in your family. You may need more frequent checks if your test results aren't in a desirable range or you have risk factors for heart disease.

- **Manage diabetes.** If you have diabetes, tight blood sugar control can help reduce the risk of heart disease.

- Physical activity helps you achieve and maintain a healthy weight. Regular exercise helps control diabetes, high cholesterol, and high blood pressure—all risk factors for heart disease. With your provider's OK, aim for 30 to 60 minutes of physical activity most days of the week. Talk to your health care provider about the amount and type of exercise that's best for you.

- **Maintain a healthy weight.** Being overweight increases the risk of heart disease. Talk with your care provider to set realistic goals for body mass index (BMI) and weight.

- **Manage stress.** Find ways to help reduce emotional stress. Getting more exercise, practicing mindfulness, and connecting with others in support groups are some ways to reduce and manage stress. If you have anxiety or depression, talk to your provider about strategies to help.

- **Practice good hygiene.** Regularly wash your hands and brush and floss your teeth to keep yourself healthy.

- **Practice good sleep habits.** Poor sleep may increase the risk of heart disease and other chronic conditions. Adults should aim to get 7 to 9 hours of sleep daily. Kids often need more. Go to bed and wake up at the same time every day, including on weekends.

Things that you and your health care professional can do for heart disease can be all over the map, from CPR to high-tech surgeries to caregiving. Chances are that you, or someone you love, may need different types.

1. Interventions

1. Stents

A stent is a tiny tube that can play a big role in treating your heart disease. It helps keep your arteries—the blood vessels that carry blood from your heart to other parts of your body, including the heart muscle itself.

2. Angioplasty and Stents

Angioplasty is a procedure to open narrowed or blocked blood vessels that supply blood to the heart. These blood vessels are called the coronary arteries. A coronary artery stent is a small, metal mesh tube that expands inside a coronary artery. A stent is often placed during or immediately after angioplasty.

3. Heart bypass surgery

Coronary artery bypass surgery creates a new path for blood to flow around a blocked or partially blocked artery in the heart. The surgery involves taking a healthy blood vessel from the chest or leg area. The vessel is connected below the blocked heart artery. The new pathway improves blood flow to the heart muscle.

4. Valve disease treatment

Medicine, or surgery to repair or replace the valve. Treatment varies depending on the type of heart valve disease.

5. Pacemakers

Pacemakers send electrical pulses to help your heart beat at a normal rate and rhythm. Pacemakers can also be used to help your heart chambers beat in sync so your heart can pump blood more efficiently to your body. This may be needed if you have heart failure.

6. Implantable Cardioverter Defibrillators (ICD)

An implantable cardioverter-defibrillator (ICD) is a small battery-powered device placed in the chest. It detects and stops irregular heartbeats, also called arrhythmias. An ICD continuously checks the heartbeat. It delivers electric shocks when needed to restore a regular heart rhythm.

7. Lead Extraction

Lead extraction is a procedure to remove heart device leads. You may need this procedure if the leads become infected, broken, or defective. Lead extraction is a complex procedure due to the scar tissue that holds the leads in place.

8. Left Ventricular Assist Device (LVAD)

Is a pump that we use for patients who have reached end-stage heart failure?

9. Heart Transplant

A heart transplant is a treatment that's usually reserved for people whose condition hasn't improved enough with medications or other treatments.

10. Drug-Eluting Stents

Are vascular prostheses used by interventional cardiologists to reopen and maintain patent coronary arteries narrowed by arteriosclerosis?

2. **Medications**

1. ACE Inhibitors

2. Angiotension II receptor blockers

3. Antiarrhythmics

4. Antiplatelet Drugs

5. Aspirin Therapy

6. Beta-Blocker Therapy

7. Calcium Channel Blocker Drugs

8. Clot-buster drugs

9. Nitrates

10. How to Take Heart Medication

3. Care

1. Recovery After Heart Surgery

2. Finding Strength During Tough Times

Although you might know that eating certain foods can increase your heart disease risk, changing your eating habits is often tough. Whether you have years of unhealthy eating under your belt or you simply want to fine-tune your diet, here are eight heart-healthy diet tips. Once you know which foods to eat more of and which foods to limit, you'll be on your way towards a heart-healthy diet.

1. **Control your portion size.**

How much you eat is just as important as what you eat. Overloading your plate, taking seconds, and eating until you feel stuffed can lead to eating more calories than you should. Portions served in restaurants are often more than anyone needs.

Following a few simple tips to control food portion size can help you shape up your diet as well as your heart and waistline:

- Use a small plate or bowl to help control your portions.

- Eat more low-calorie, nutrient-rich foods, such as fruits and vegetables.

- Eat smaller amounts of high-calorie, high-sodium foods, such as refined, processed, or fast foods.

It's also important to keep track of the number of servings you eat. Some things to keep in mind:

- A serving size is a specific amount of food, defined by common measurements such as cups, ounces, or pieces. For example, one serving of pasta is about 1/3 to 1/2 cup, or about the size of a hockey puck. A serving of meat, fish, or chicken is about 2 to 3 ounces, or about the size and thickness of a deck of cards.

- The recommended number of servings per food group may vary depending on the specific diet or guidelines you're following.

- Judging serving size is a learned skill. You may need to use measuring cups and spoons or a scale until you're comfortable with your judgement.

2. **Eat more vegetables and fruits.**

Vegetables and fruits are good sources of vitamins and minerals. Vegetables and fruits are also low in calories and rich in dietary fiber. Vegetables and fruits, like other plants or plant-based foods, contain substances that may help prevent cardiovascular disease. Eating more fruits and vegetables may help you cut back on higher-calorie foods, such as meat, cheese, and snack foods.

Including vegetables and fruits in your diet can be easy. Keep vegetables washed and cut in your refrigerator for quick snacks. Keep fruit in a bowl in your kitchen so that you'll remember to eat it. Choose recipes that have vegetables or fruits as the main ingredients, such as vegetable stir-fry or fresh fruit mixed into salads.

3. **Select whole grains.**

Whole grains are good sources of fibre and other nutrients that play a role in regulating blood pressure and heart health. You can increase the amount of whole grains in a heart-healthy diet by making simple substitutions for refined grain products. Or be adventurous and try a new whole grain, such as whole-grain farro, quinoa, or barley.

4. **Limit unhealthy fats.**

Limiting how much saturated and trans fat you eat is an important step to reducing your blood cholesterol and lowering your risk of coronary artery disease. A high blood cholesterol level can lead to a buildup of plaques in the arteries, called atherosclerosis, which can increase the risk of heart attack and stroke.

5. **Choose low-fat protein sources'**

Lean meat, poultry and fish, low-fat dairy products, and eggs are some of the best sources of protein. Choose lower-fat options, such as skinless chicken breasts rather than fried chicken patties, and skim milk rather than whole milk.

Fish is a good alternative to high-fat meats. Certain types of fish are rich in omega-3 fatty acids, which can lower blood fats called triglycerides. You'll find the highest amounts of omega-3 fatty acids in cold-water fish, such as salmon, mackerel, and herring. Other sources are flaxseed, walnuts, soybeans, and canola oil.

Legumes—beans, peas, and lentils—are also good, low-fat sources of protein and contain no cholesterol, making them good substitutes for meat. Substituting plant protein for animal protein—for example, a soy or bean burger for a hamburger—will reduce fat and cholesterol intake and increase fibre intake.

6. **Reduce salt (sodium).)**

Eating too much salt can lead to high blood pressure, a risk factor for heart disease. Limiting salt (sodium) is an important part of a heart-healthy diet. The American Heart Association recommends that:

- Healthy adults have no more than 2,300 milligrams (mg) of sodium a day (about a teaspoon of salt).

- Most adults ideally have no more than 1,500 mg of sodium a day.

Although reducing the amount of salt you add to food at the table or while cooking is a good first step, much of the salt you eat comes from canned or processed foods, such as soups, baked goods, and frozen dinners. Eating fresh foods and making your own soups and stews can reduce the amount of salt you eat.

If you like the convenience of canned soups and prepared meals, look for ones with no added salt or reduced sodium. Be wary of foods that claim to be lower in sodium because they are seasoned with sea salt instead of regular table salt; sea salt has the same nutritional value as regular salt.

Another way to reduce the amount of salt you eat is to choose your condiments carefully. Many condiments are available in reduced-sodium versions. Salt substitutes can add flavor to your food with less sodium.

7. **Plan ahead: Create daily menus.**

Create daily menus using the six strategies listed above. When selecting foods for each meal and snack, emphasize vegetables, fruits, and whole grains. Choose lean protein sources and healthy fats, and limit salty foods. Watch your portion sizes and add variety to your menu choices.

For example, if you have grilled salmon one evening, try a black bean burger the next night. This helps ensure that you'll get all of the nutrients your body needs. Variety also makes meals and snacks more interesting.

8. **Allow yourself an occasional treat.**

Allow yourself an indulgence every now and then. A candy bar or handful of potato chips won't derail your heart-healthy diet. But don't let it turn into an excuse for giving up on your healthy eating plan. If overindulgence is the exception rather than the rule, you'll balance things out over the long term. What's important is that you eat healthy foods most of the time.

Include these eight tips in your life, and you'll find that heart-healthy eating is both doable and enjoyable. With planning and a few simple substitutions, you can eat with your heart in mind.

Natural Remedies

But is there a faster way to give your heart an extra boost? Swipe your digital device or turn on the TV, and you'll see ad after ad for natural remedies that can heal your heart and help you live longer. But do they work? A panel of heart doctors and pharmacists takes a look at some common herbal supplements and tells you which ones work and which ones are just hype.

Garlic

Garlic's been used for centuries to boost heart health, among other things. When you crush it, you release a compound called allicin. It's what gives garlic its stinky odor. Scientists think it helps keep your arteries flexible and let's blood flow better. "There are numerous, well-documented studies on garlic and its benefit to cardiovascular health," says David Foreman, RPh, author of 4 Pillars of Health: Heart Disease. "It helps lower cholesterol, blood pressure, and inflammation. This combined effect can help decrease the risk of both heart attacks and strokes."

Coenzyme Q-10 (CoQ10)

If you take drugs to lower your cholesterol (and have muscle pain as a side effect), doctors agree an antioxidant called CoQ10 may be worth a try. It's found naturally in nearly every body tissue, including the heart. It helps your cells make the energy they need to grow.

Red Yeast Rice

Need to lower your cholesterol but don't want to take a prescription drug? Boyden recommends this ancient remedy made by mixing fermented rice with yeast.

"It's a naturopathic statin," he says. "It actually was the genesis for one of the very first statins, and there is good evidence to support it."

Flaxseed

Here's another natural option for helping keep your cholesterol in check: But if you're at high risk, you probably shouldn't take it in place of your medication.

Flaxseed is rich in omega-3 fatty acids, which is often a heart-healthy diet choice. Omega-3s help lower blood pressure and inflammation. They also contain fibre-rich plant compounds called lignans that have been shown to reduce cholesterol and plaque buildup in the arteries.

To get the most benefit for your heart, choose the seeds, not the oil. "The seeds should be ground, milled, and preferably fresh in order to impact health," Foreman says. "If not, the whole seed will pass through the body without being digested, like corn, and yield zero health benefits."

Vitamin K2

Vitamin K2 is frequently linked to better heart health. A 2014 study showed that diets rich in vitamin K (think of leafy, green veggies) helped reduce the risk of death due to heart problems in people who were at high risk for the disease.

"It helps prevent calcium in the bloodstream from depositing in the arteries and blood vessels," says Dennis Goodman, author of Vitamin K2: The Missing Nutrient for Heart and Bone Health.

Scientists think people who don't get enough vitamin K2 have more calcium deposits in their arteries and a higher risk for heart disease. "Keeping calcium in bone and out of the arteries results in improved blood vessel function and reduces age-related stiffness of the arteries," Goodman adds.

Clinical studies are underway to see if vitamin K2 can help reduce blockages leading to heart attacks and strokes.

If you want to keep your heart healthy, you'll typically do three things: choose nutritious foods, stay active, and toss bad habits like smoking.

To keep your spirits up:

- Get dressed every day.

- Walk daily.

- Pick up your hobbies and social activities.

- Share your feelings with others.

- Get a good night's sleep.

Limit visits to 15 minutes at first. As you feel stronger and less tired, spend more time with your visitors.

Rest and sleep.

Many people have trouble sleeping after heart surgery. You should get back to a normal slumber pattern within a few months.

If pain keeps you up, take medication about half an hour before bedtime. Arrange the pillows so you can stay in a comfortable position.

You'll probably need to rest after an activity, but try not to take a lot of naps during the day.

In the evening, avoid caffeine includes chocolate, coffee, tea, and some sodas. Settle into a bedtime routine, perhaps listening to relaxing music. Your body will learn that these cues mean it's time to snooze.

The three main things you should do to maintain heart health are to eat well, be active, and give up harmful habits like smoking.

Is there, however, a quicker method to give your heart a boost? You'll see advertisement after advertisement for all-natural cures that may strengthen your heart and lengthen your life if you swipe your digital gadget or turn on the TV.

You can use this guide to help you make healthier choices when:

.planning what to eat

.cooking or preparing a meal at home

.food shopping

eating out or on the go

Most of the meals we eat are a combination of food groups. When planning meals, work out the main ingredients and think about how these fit within the 5 main food groups.